Gerontology

Books of related interest

Ageing, Independence and the Life Course
Edited by Sara Arber and Maria Evandrou
ISBN 1 85302 180 6

The Abuse of Elderly People
A Handbook for Professionals
Jacki Pritchard
ISBN 1 85302 122 9

The Psychology of Ageing
An Introduction
Ian Stuart-Hamilton
ISBN 1 85302 063 X

Gerontology

Responding to an Ageing Society

Edited by Kevin Morgan

Jessica Kingsley Publishers in association with
The British Society of Gerontology

Acknowledgements

In preparing this reader I have been supported both by the contributors, and the Publications Committee of the British Society of Gerontology. My thanks to the former for their patience and co-operation, and to the latter for providing a reliable source of encouragement and guidance. Thanks also to Hazel Binks for downloading and preparing the original contributions. As a particularly slow reader, I am grateful for the help given by my colleagues in the Department of Health Care of the Elderly, Jeanette Lilley, Kate Bennett, and Roger Rumble, in checking and amending the text. Finally, special thanks to Jennifer Brookes for her advice and skilled assistance throughout the editing of the manuscript.

First published in the United Kingdom in 1992 by
Jessica Kingsley Publishers Ltd
116 Pentonville Road
London N1 9JB
in association with The British Society of Gerontology

British Library Cataloguing in Publication Data
Gerontology: Responding to an Ageing
Society
I. Morgan, Kevin
362.6

ISBN 1-85302-117-2

Printed and bound in Great Britain by
Biddles Ltd, Guildford and King's Lynn

Contents

List of Figures

Tables

Contributors

Sara Arber — Senior Lecturer,
Department of Sociology,
University of Surrey,
Guildford, Surrey GU2 5XH.

Simon Biggs — Programme Coordinator,
Community Care Programme,
Central Council for Education and
Training in Social Work,
Derbyshire House,
St Chad's Street,
London WC1H 8AD
and:
Fellow of the Centre for Social Gerontology,
University of Keele, ST5 5BG

Michael Carley — Senior Research Fellow,
Policy Studies Institute,
100 Park Village East,
London NW1 3SR.

Tim Dant — Senior Lecturer in Sociology
Department of Social Science,
Manchester Polytechnic
Chatham / Undercroft Building,
Cavendish Street,
Manchester M15 6BR.

Bleddyn Davies — Director,
Personal Social Services Research Unit, Cornwallis Building,
The University ,
Canterbury,
Kent CT2 7NF.

Shah Ebrahim — Professor and Head of Department,
Joint Department of Health Care of the Elderly,
London Hospital Medical College,
The London Hospital (Mile End),
Bancroft Road, London E1 4DG.

Brian Gearing — Senior Lecturer in Health and Social Welfare
Department of Health and Social Welfare,
The Open University, Walton Hall,
Milton Keynes MK7 6AA.

Chris Gilleard — Top Grade Clinical Psychologist
and Senior Lecturer in the Psychology of Old Age,
Springfield University Hospital and St Georges Hospital Medical School,
Tooting, London SW17 7DJ.

Jay Ginn — Research Officer,
Department of Sociology,
University of Surrey,
Guildford, Surrey GU2 5XH.

Silvana di Gregorio	Lecturer in Social Policy, School of Management Cranfield Institute of Technology, Cranfield, Bedford MK40 0AL.
Paul Higgs	Eleanor Peel Lecturer in Gerontology, Department of Geriatric Medicine, St Georges Hospital Medical School, University of London, Level 01, Jenner Wing G2, Cranmer Terrace, Tooting, London SW17 0RE.
Malcolm Johnson	Professor and Director, Institute of Health and Social Welfare and Community Education The Open University, Walton Hall, Milton Keynes MK7 6AA.
Ian R. Jones	Research Fellow in Healthcare Needs, The Health Care Research Unit, Queen Mary and Westfield College, University of London, Mile End, London E1 4NS.
Anthea Lehmann	Consultant Geriatrician, Department of Geriatric Medicine, St Bartholomew's Hospital, West Smithfield, London EC1A 7BE.
Kevin Morgan	Lecturer in Gerontology, Department of Health Care of the Elderly, University of Nottingham Medical School, Nottingham NG7 2UH.
Ann Netten	Research Fellow, Personal Social Services Research Unit, Cornwallis Building, The University, Canterbury, Kent CT2 7NF.
Christopher W. Smith	Senior Lecturer in Geography, Thames Valley University, St Mary's Road, Ealing, London W5 5RF.
Anthony M. Warnes,	Professor of Geography and Research Associate, Age Concern Institute of Gerontology, King's College London, Cornwall House, Waterloo Road London SE1 8TX.
Alexandra Withnall,	Senior Research Officer, Office of Adult Continuing Education, University of Lancaster, Cartmel College, Lancaster LA1 4YL.

CHAPTER 1

Introduction

Kevin Morgan

Like the people it measures and describes gerontology itself has, in recent years, taken several important steps towards maturity. The increasing prominence given to ageing issues in the training of health and social service professionals, the growth of specialised post-graduate courses, and the continued expansion of gerontological research and literature all indicate the importance now attached to this once neglected and marginalised topic.

Among the many factors contributing to this state of affairs, and one of the notable features of any large gerontological convention or conference, is the sheer breadth of interest now being shown in both ageing individuals, and ageing societies. Practitioners, policy-makers, and researchers from a variety of backgrounds currently share a sense of common purpose around the theme of human ageing. Whether the result is conceptualised as a discipline or a confederation of disciplinary interests, it is important to recognise that one of the strengths of contemporary gerontology lies in its eclecticism.

Underpinning this eclectic interest in ageing research is a marked and general shift towards pragmatism. Social gerontology has moved from its lengthy concern with functionalist theory towards a more practical involvement in the social ecology of elderly people. Psychological gerontology has largely abandoned its early self-appointed role of 'counting and classifying the wrinkles of aged behavior' (Kastenbaum 1968, pp.280–283), and tends now to be more concerned with the implications of, or the circumstances which optimize that behaviour. Similar trends are identifiable within the clinical sciences where the growth of old-age specialisation (Besdine 1989, pp.181–182), and the reciprocal increase in research funding, clearly testify to the new status afforded to older people as patients or as clients. Appropriately, then, the practical and intellectual issues provoked by an ageing society have become the priorities of gerontological research.

It is these two characteristics of gerontological research – eclecticism and pragmatism – which provide the over-arching theme for this reader. Broadly the book has two broad aims. First, to provide a – overview of how contemporary gerontological research is identifying and responding to the issues facing our ageing society. And second, to examine the range of approaches, methodologies, and controversies within that gerontological response.

Importantly, then, this is not a book on research devoted mainly to research findings (although of course outcome and findings are given some prominence). Neither is it intended as the gerontological equivalent of a Victorian zoo, with a single lonely animal from each species metaphorically represented in a collection of disparate chapters. Rather, it is a book concerned with the *process* of gerontological research, from the appropriate conceptualisation of research issues, through the practicalities of 'finding out', to the problems of translating research into practice. While chapters vary in approach and emphasis, each is concerned with identifying and clarifying *need*.

Within this context, 'need' can range from the support needs of elderly people living at home, to the training needs of professionals working with elderly people, or even the need to understand better some of the assumptions underlying commonly accepted views of age-related illness and health.

Though rapidly maturing, gerontology is nevertheless a relatively immature enterprise. Methodologies are still under review, ideas are still under discussion, and some outcomes are still under suspicion. (All of which provides a stimulating and necessary intellectual milieu). Furthermore, and again as a function of the relative neglect of ageing matters in the past, basic background research has yet to be done, or completed in many areas. For these reasons many of the contributions to this reader provide a point of departure, assessing what has gone before, and then describing current research steps into a given area. Where there is no established research pedigree, no obvious route to continue along the existing research can at least provide a useful theoretical framework within which to work. Overall, then, each contribution is whole in itself, introducing the topic and describing or discussing appropriate responses.

As regards the organisation of the book, no attempt has been made to cluster semantically any of the chapters. The reasons for this are obvious enough given the emphasis on eclecticism. Clustering according to topic (e.g. economics, residential care, community care) would have produced one sequence, while discipline (psychology, human geography, medicine) would have produced another, and approach (biographical, qualitative, national statistics) a third, etc. Instead, the principle influences on chapter order have been either aesthetic, or subliminal.

References

Besdine, R.W. (1989) The maturing of geriatrics. *New England Journal of Medicine* 320, 181-182.

Kastenbaum, R. (1968) Perspectives on the development and modification of behavior in the aged: A developmental-field perspective. *The Gerontologist* 8, 280-283.

CHAPTER 2

Elderly People Driving Cars
Issues and Prospects

Anthony M. Warnes

This chapter examines the implications of the growing use of private cars as a means of transport among elderly people. The growth is primarily a reflection of growing affluence and the chronology of private motorisation and has only a weak association with changes in a nation's age structure. In many western European countries, those born in the 1930s and later have been the first cohorts to experience majority car ownership from early adulthood and to bring driving skills and habitual dependence upon cars into old age. An awareness of the multiplication of older drivers has recently developed in road transport circles and older people's organisations. Some have been concerned with the safety of older drivers; others with the mobility difficulties faced by people who have to give up cars. But with the exception of research in cognitive psychology, driving has received little attention from gerontologists.

The paper opens with the problems of describing, interpreting and forecasting the spread of car ownership and use among the older population. Later sections consider several applied issues for elderly people and for society, including the benefits and problems of car dependency, the limitations of old people as drivers, and the implications of a rising complement of older people among drivers for transport policy, traffic regulations and drivers' behaviour. What are the implications for both those with and without the use of cars?

The Growth of Car Ownership and Use

The timing of the spread of private car ownership has been influenced in different countries by their economic growth and settlement characteristics. Car dependency among elderly people is highest in North America where demographic ageing is less advanced than in North West Europe. Mass car ownership came about during the second quarter of this century in the United States, during the third quarter in northern Europe and two decades later (and so is now at its peak rate of increase) in Portugal, Spain and Greece (Thomson 1977). A moderating influence has been the competitiveness of alternative forms of transport (including walking). Travel needs have been satisfied more comprehensively without private cars in European cities than in low density American urban areas or in rural areas in all countries.

Car ownership and use among the older population of the United States and Canada have recently reached very high levels. The share with licences among those aged 65+ years increased in the USA from 43% in 1969 to 62% in 1983 and in Canada from 31% in 1967 to 50% in 1982 (USA Committee for the Study on Improving Mobility and Safety for Older Persons 1988; OECD 1985, Table III.5). There are strong sex differentials. In 1983 in the USA, four out of five elderly men but slightly fewer than half of the elderly women held licences. The most rural, recently developed and prosperous regions of the United States have the highest rates of motorisation. In California in 1982, 64% of the 65+ years population had driving licences and, among those aged 80+ years, 58% of men and 18% of women held licences (California Department of Motor Vehicles 1982). In January 1990 in Florida, 90% of men aged 65+ years and 68% of women held licences (Florida Department of Highway Safety and Motor Vehicles 1990).

By 1989 levels of licence holding among elderly males in England and Wales were similar to those of the United States while the female rate, although growing fast, remained significantly lower (Figure 2.1). The age/sex groups which showed the greatest changes in licence holding

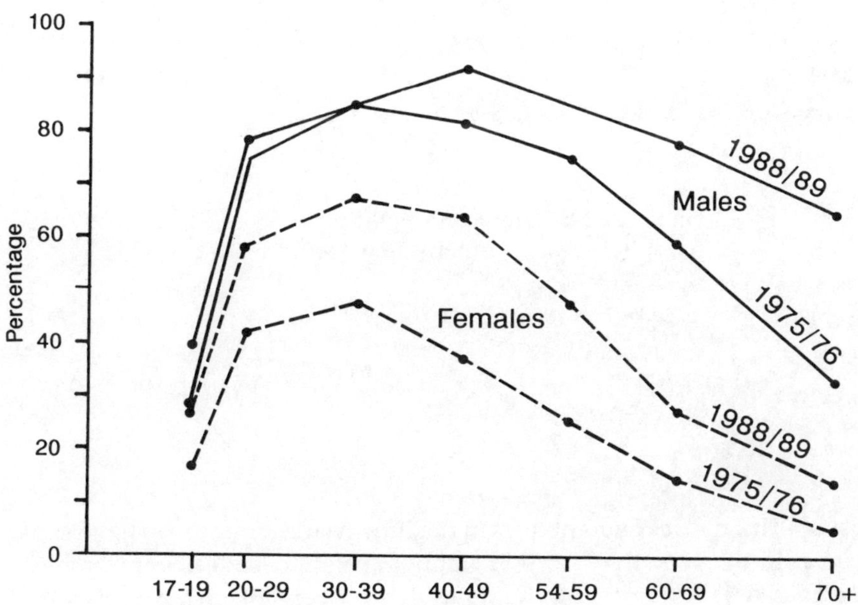

Figure 2.1: Levels of licence holding among men and women in England and Wales (1975/76 and 1988/89;)

between 1975/76 and 1988/89 were males aged 50+ and women aged 30–59 years. Among women aged 70+ years the licence holding rate almost tripled to 14%.

Table 2.1 Rates of household car ownership: England and Wales and the London Metropolitan Region, 1981

	England & Wales %	*Greater London County* %	*Outer Metropol-itan Area* %	*Outer South East* %	*Ratio to England & Wales* GLC	OMA	OSE
All households	61.5	55.3	73.5	66.8	0.90	1.19	1.09
Households with 1+pensioner	39.0	34.6	47.6	44.9	0.89	1.22	1.15
Single person households							
Males 65–74 years	32.0	25.9	42.7	41.2	0.81	1.33	1.29
Males 75+ years	17.7	13.5	21.8	23.9	0.76	1.23	1.35
Females 60–74 years	14.0	10.9	19.0	20.3	0.78	1.36	1.45
Females 75+ years	5.0	3.8	6.8	7.8	0.76	1.36	1.56
Two or more pensioner households							
All <75 years	55.0	48.8	64.3	64.7	0.89	1.17	1.18
1+ aged 75+ years	33.8	26.8	39.4	41.0	0.79	1.17	1.21

Source: Office of Population Censuses and Surveys (1983) Table 8.

Table 2.2 Driving licence holding by age (%), West Germany 1976–2000

	Males			*Females*		
Age Group	*1976*	*1985*	*2000*	*1976*	*1985*	*2000*
60–69	57	72	90	12	25	50
70–79	25	53	80	3	11	30
80–89	7	21	65	1	2	17

Source: OECD (1985).

Most of Britain's near neighbours in the European Community have experienced a similar growth of car ownership in recent decades. Some have seen faster increases in association with rapid improvements in living standards. At present, less than one quarter of all persons aged 60+ years are licensed drivers in the member nations, but Table 2.2 shows that in West Germany by the end of the century, near universal male licensing is expected and female licence holding will be growing very fast (OECD 1985).

An alternative measure of car dependency is the household possession of cars. Data from the 1981 England and Wales population census demonstrates the strong variations by income, sex, age, household composition and urban/rural area of residence (Table 2.1). Whereas 61.5% of all households possessed at least one car, only 39% of households with pensioners did so. Among pensioner households, ownership rates varied by age, sex and household size. Fifty-five per cent of 2+ person young pensioner households possessed cars, but only 5% of 75+ years single woman households. Table 2.1 presents comparable rates for the erstwhile Greater London County (GLC) area, the Outer Metropolitan Area (OMA; around London up to approximately 30km from the centre), and the Outer South East (which includes the coastal retirement towns of Essex, Kent and Sussex). The data illustrate the universal phenomenon of low car ownership in cities and high rural ownership rates. In the GLC, household car ownership was generally 10% lower than in the country while in the OMA it was 20% higher. The variations are greater among pensioner than younger households. Ownership rates among single pensioners aged 75+ years were 24% lower in London than in England and Wales and, for females, 56% higher in the Outer South East.

Car Driving by Age and Sex

Detailed series on age-specific driving licence holding and car ownership are available from several affluent countries. In England and Wales, licence holding rates climb from the late teen-ages to people in their thirties or early forties after which they fall approximately linearly (Figure 2.1). Among males in 1988/89, the rate peaks at 92% among those aged 40–49 years and falls to 62% among those aged 70+ years. The female rates are considerably lower, the peak being 67% among those aged 30–39 years, with a fall to 14% among those aged 70+ years. Since 1975, the peak rates have tended to shift to the right and the late-age gradient has become less steep.

The comparable series for Florida show broadly similar forms except that the peak rates of licence holding are among people in their twenties (Figure 2.2). In fact they exceed 100% of the population, probably caused by out-of-State registrants including students. In 1989 the population licence holding rate declined exponentially after the age of 30 years to around 80% by the early fifties, and fluctuated around this level at older ages to the early seventies. By January 1990 among those aged 65+ years, nine in ten men and two-thirds (67.6%) of women held licences (Figure 2.3) (Florida Department of Highway Safety and Motor Vehicles 1990). Even allowing that in the United States licences are retained as surrogate identity cards by those who have given up driving, eg to cash cheques at supermarkets, the high rates of possession among men and the absence of an age-related decline before 85+ years is striking (Eisenhandler 1990). One local factor must be the paucity of alternatives to the private car in almost all counties of Florida. Older people

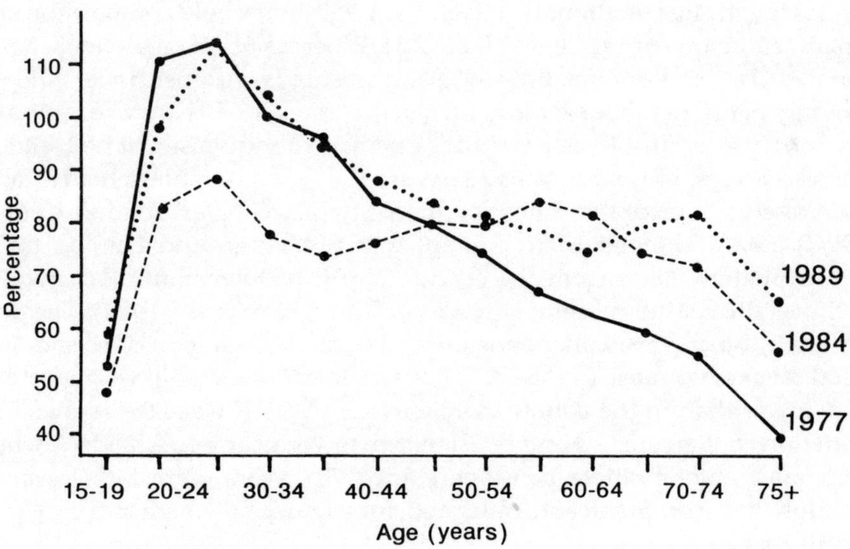

Figure 2.2 : Levels of licence holding in Florida, USA (1977, 1984, and 1989)

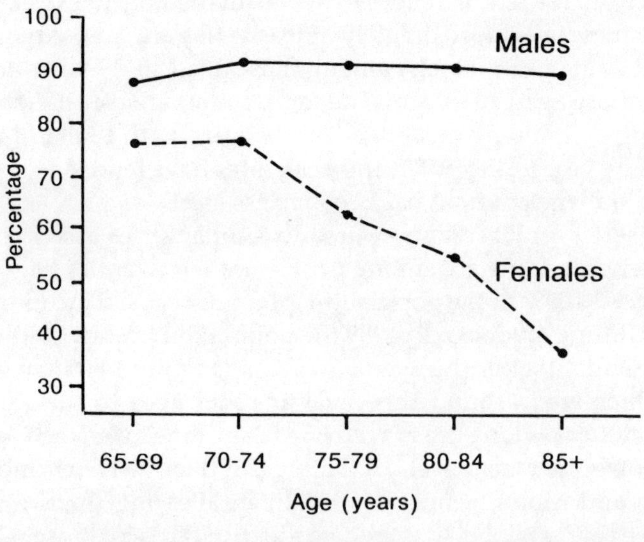

Figure 2.3 : Levels of licence holding in Florida, USA (January 1990)

in the State without the use of cars face considerable travel inconvenience and restriction.

Technological Innovation and Age-Patterns of Adoption

The protracted adoption of car use by elderly people has less to do with demographic ageing than with the history of motor vehicle development and use during this century. The diffusion illustrates some general features of the adoption of new technologies and social forms. At least three conditions have been required for cars to become a mass form of transport: sufficient advances in vehicle design and manufacturing processes to reduce the real cost of ownership and use (partly through improved reliability and lower maintenance costs); sufficient personal incomes; and the widespread possession of driving skills. The economic history of the car market is less relevant to this paper than the diffusion of driving skills.

At present, the decision to learn to drive is normally secondary to those which make a private car available. The two transitions were formerly less clearly linked. During the last 70 years, many middle-aged and older people have had the means to purchase a private car but have lacked driving skills and been unable or insufficiently motivated to learn. In Britain, many men born before the 1930s who learnt to drive did so on commercial vehicles, as motor-cyclists, or in the armed services during the Second World War. Women had many fewer opportunities to learn. Moreover, the strong differentiation of marriage roles, and the car's prime value for journeys to and from work (except in the largest cities), also retarded women's access to cars. The recent convergence of male and female economic activity rates and sex-role norms have therefore reinforced rising affluence in encouraging multiple household car-ownership and in reducing the male-female differential in driving licensing.

The Launch Phase

Concepts from historical epidemiology and theories of the diffusion of technological innovations throw light on the spread of driving. Its incidence is represented by the age and sex of learners and its prevalence by the characteristics of licentiates or, less perfectly, car owners. Each innovation adoption process shares generic features as well as patterns specific to itself (Hagerstrand 1967; Rogers 1983). There must first be a 'launch' phase, when the gender and age characteristics of adopters are distinctive. If an innovation becomes available to a mass market over a short period (say less than ten years), persons of all ages are likely to adopt. Once the innovation has saturated the population, however, further adoptions will be concentrated among young people. The ages of first purchasers of automatic washing machines and of new telephone subscribers must have changed in this manner from the 1950s to the present. Every innovation shows variations in

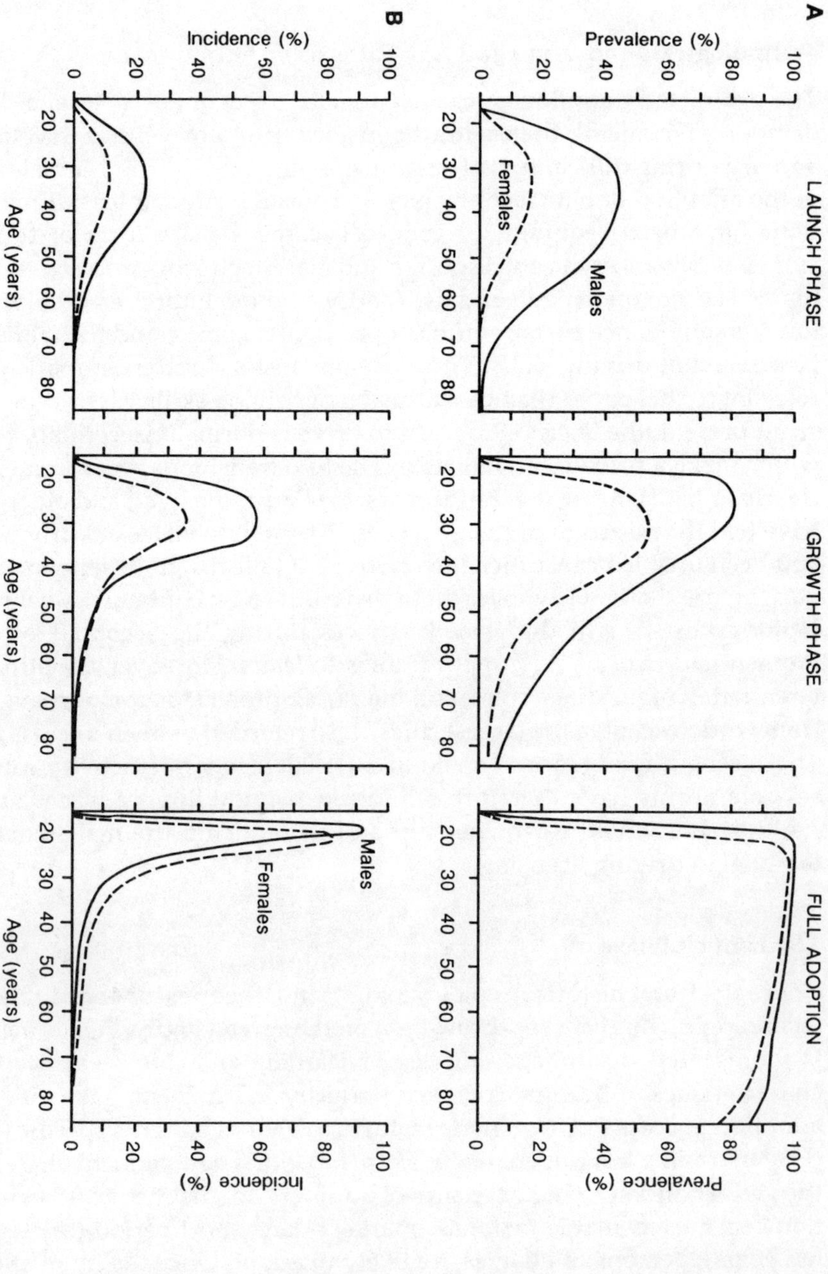

Figure 2.4: The adoption of car use by age and historical phase

adoption according to its technological and economic characteristics, ie its function, complexity and price. Age-selectivity among early drivers arose for three reasons: the skill involves adult responsibility and most countries quickly introduced licensing which excluded minors; a high proportion of vehicles in the growth phase were commercial (trucks, buses, taxis) favouring men of middle-working ages; and, most importantly, strong selectivity by income and socioeconomic group applied. The first learners in most countries would have been adult men of all ages with a probable bias towards middle age produced by both income and occupational seniority effects (Figure 2.4).

Age-selectivity in early private car ownership was more directly controlled by the income effect. The high price of motor cars exaggerated the normal phenomenon of products being most costly during their launch phase, with the consequence that early adopters were of high income. A moderating influence would have been differential utility. Even in the launch phase, car ownership in rural areas was higher than in towns.

The Growth Phase

A growth phase follows the launch. In the case of driving in Britain, this has extended over more than half a century. Early in the growth phase, high rates of learning and licence holding are established among people in their twenties and there continue to be many 'late learners' (Figure 2.4). The starting pattern also shows pronounced male:female differences, which are greatest among the youngest and oldest adults. Over time, the concentration of learning in the earliest adult ages increases, all age-specific licentiate rates rise, the peak prevalence of licence holding moves to younger ages, and the gender differentials reduce in a wave from the youngest to the oldest age groups.

Empirical evidence for this evolution in Britain is fullest for the later stages of the growth phase. By the mid 1970s (and probably as early as the 1950s), learning to drive was concentrated among very young adults, particularly in males. In October 1974 one half of men's but only three in ten of women's driving tests were taken at less than 21 years of age (Table 2.3). By 1985, the concentration had increased to 61% and 43% respectively. In 1974, among those taking driving tests when aged 21–40 years women outnumbered men by 60%. Only 10% of men's but 17% of women's tests were of people aged more than 40 years. By 1985 the frequency of late learning had fallen to 4% of men's and 11% of women's tests. (The all-age pass rate in 1985 was 44% for females and 53% for males, resulting in a greater number of tests for women than men).

Table 2.3 Age of persons taking driving tests: England and Wales 1974–1985

	Men (%)				*Women(%)*			
Year	*<21*	*21–40*	*41–50*	*50+*	*<21*	*–40*	*41–50*	*50+*
1974	50.0	39.6	6.2	4.2	28.9	53.8	11.5	5.8
1980	58.7	34.8	4.3	2.2	38.9	48.1	7.4	5.6
1985	60.9	34.8	4.3		42.5	48.1	11.1	

Note: Figures are based on sample surveys, in 1974 of all motor car tests conducted on two days in October. The 1980 survey was also conducted in October and the 1985 survey in April.

Source: Department of Transport (1976) Table 60; Department of Transport (1990) Table 2.18.

Full Adoption

The growth phase ends with saturation adoption, first of licence holding and, after a long lag, of independent car access, which is unlikely to become so pervasive. Almost all Floridian men have driving licences: their age-prevalence schedule shows no decline before age 80 years. This pattern can be hypothesised as the final schedule for both sexes in all countries. Among women in Florida, however, licence holding among elderly women is still increasing and still declines with age in later life. Occupational and income inequalities will probably preserve the differential for many decades. Elsewhere in the United States and throughout Europe, substantial scope remains for the further spread of driving skills and car access.

Cars as Facilitators of Activities

Until recently cars have had a small role in enabling the activity patterns of elderly people. As a noted study 20 years ago in San Antonio, Texas commented, 'the low incidence of unrestricted driving on the part of retirees has serious implications in a society so highly geared to the automobile. For the sizable majority who do not drive, transportation problems may severely limit all aspects of life during the retirement years' (Carp 1972, 788). Most studies in social gerontology of travel and transport have emphasised the reliance of elderly people upon walking, lifts (car passenger journeys) and on public transport (Markovitz 1971; Norman 1977; Robson 1982). The problems of transport availability, cost, boarding, dismounting, carrying goods and personal safety have all been described.

An unusually comprehensive study of elderly people's personal mobility in Britain in 1971–72 found that few pensioners had access to cars, that the age group was highly dependent on walking and buses, that their travel purposes were dominated by shopping and social trips, and that a large proportion (41%) had difficulties with walking in their local areas (Hillman, Henderson and Whalley 1976). Survey evidence from the numerous 1960s/1970s regional and metropolitan transportation studies suggested that the diversity of personal travel patterns could be classified into three groups on the basis of journey purposes, modes, distances and diurnal patterns: those undertaken by (i) children and students; (ii) working-age males and full-time employed women; and (iii) housewives, part-time employed women and the retired (Daniels and Warnes 1980, 36–52). The third group's trips were (and no doubt still are) distinguished by low mean aggregate trip distances, few work-related journeys, a relative predominance of shopping, personal business and social trips, and a broad spread of trips from mid-morning until early evening with relatively few in the morning peak.

The 1985/86 GB National Travel Survey provides a recent profile of elderly people's travel. Their weekly travel distance was 58% that of working-age women and 35% that of working-age men. The differentials are associated with car ownership and work travel. Half the elderly population were in households with cars and a third were licensed drivers, but only 16% of those living alone owned cars. Continued employment is a spur to car ownership and a high travel distance (Table 2.4). 'Single adult households were less likely than larger households to be car-owners, even allowing for their lower incomes. Elderly single person households (80% of whom were in the lowest income quartile) had few cars but, after adjusting for income, other single adult households were only slightly less likely to have a car' (Department of Transport 1988, 27).

Table 2.4 Car ownership by age and household group: United Kingdom 1985/86

	Households with cars		*Cars per household*	
	%	*Adjusted %**	%	*Adjusted %**
Single adult households				
<60years	16	52	0.16	0.52
60+ years	43	56	0.46	0.60
Two person households				
Both <60 years	80	68	1.06	0.87
1+ 60+ years	61	68	0.70	0.84
All households	62	62	0.83	0.83

Note: * Controlled for income of household group
Source: Department of Transport (1988) Tables 5.5 and 5.11

Elderly people made 1.7 bus journeys each week in 1985/86 during which they travelled 5.9 miles, more than children or working-age men (Table 2.5). Their use of buses has declined in the last 20 years, but less than other age groups. Elderly people make more short (<1 mile) walking journeys than working-age males but significantly fewer than children and younger women, and they make fewer longer walking trips than all other groups. Elderly women walk overall 4 miles per week, elderly men 5 miles, and all

Table 2.5. Personal travel distances per week (miles) by purpose, mode, age and sex: United Kingdom 1985/86

	Car access		*Purposes*			*Modes*			
	Main drivers	*No car h'holds*	*Work*	*Personal business*	*Leisure*	*Bus 1985*	*Bus Change%*	*Walk*	*All*
Children	–	24	9	15	33	4.5	-44#	5.6	57
Males 16–59	211	64	85	26	52	5.0	-62#	5.3	163
Females 16–59	153	49	25	28	47	7.0	-54#	5.9	100
Elderly people	110	31	7	19	32	5.9	-34#	4.4	58
All	177	41	35	23	42	5.7	-52#	5.4	100

Note: # Percentage change in bus mileage 1965 to 1985/86
Source: Department of Transport (1988) Tables 2.4, 4.6, 7.6 and 8.3

others 5.6 miles (Department of Transport 1988, Tables 8.3 and 8.9). The purposes of elderly people's journeys were distinctive, with a high prevalence of social, leisure and shopping trips.

Car dependency among elderly people in the United States is, perhaps surprisingly, greater than in younger age groups. This is explained by elderly people's infrequent work journeys to and from city centres, almost the only journey category in the USA which is well served by public transport (USA Committee for the Study on Improving Mobility and Safety for Older Persons (CSIMSOP 1988, 29). In 1983, four in five elderly persons' trips were by private car, walking being the only other significant means of transport (Table 2.6). Increasing age after 65 years is associated with a slow decline in car use, a more rapid decline of driving mileage, and a relative increase in walking. Since 1977, elderly people's, and especially very old persons', trip patterns have changed faster than those of other age groups, with a marked reduction of walking.

The American data show that car availability promotes the frequency and distance of trips, and that increasing age after 50 years is associated with

Table 2.6. Elderly persons trip mode distribution (%) in the United States 1983 and change since 1977

	Age Group (years)							
	65–74		*75–84*		*85+*		*All ages*	
Mode	*1983 %*	*83:77 ratio*	*1983 %*	*83:77 ratio*	*1983 %*	*83:77 ratio*	*1983 %*	*83:77 ratio*
Private vehicle	86.4	1.04	84.0	1.11	78.8	1.12	84.7	1.01
Public transport	2.9	0.83	2.7	0.75	3.7	0.93	2.6	0.96
Walking	9.8	0.80	12.6	0.61	13.7	0.53	8.9	0.96
Other	0.9	0.75	0.7	1.40	3.8	*	3.8	0.90

Note: * No 'other' trips recorded in 1977
Source: USA Department of Transportation (1986) cited in USA CSIMSOP (1988) Table 2.5, 29

lower annual driving mileage (15k for males aged 50–54 years to 4k at 80–84 years). There is however a positive association with car passenger mileage. The ratio of travelled to driven private car miles increases from 1.6 in the early fifties to 2.8 for the 75+ years (CSIMSOP 1988). These figures indicate the extent to which people in advanced old age become dependent upon others for their transport. Unfortunately no data have been identified to show the relative importance of rides driven by members of the same household, relatives, or friends and neighbours. Taxis and public transport are unimportant modes nationally but critical for a minority. Federally-subsidised community transport is used by a minority of very poor, car-less and solitary elderly people in the USA.

Elderly People as Vulnerable and Hazardous Road Users

There is considerable research evidence to show that with advanced age there is a decline in physical and cognitive capacities relevant to driving (Kline 1987; Planek and Overend 1973; Ponds, Brouwer and van Wolffelaar 1988; Retchin et al 1988; Taira 1989; Welford 1982). This is partly due among healthy individuals to reductions in visual functions, mental processing and psycho-motor speeds, and partly to the high prevalence of incapacities among elderly people, such as arthritis or glaucoma (Graca 1986; Reuben, Silliman and Traines 1988). These decrements are implicated in the relatively high accident rates of elderly drivers per unit distance of driving, although it should be emphasised that their period accident rate is low (OECD 1985). In the United States, persons aged 65+ years comprise 11% of all drivers but only 4% of drivers in fatal accidents and 2% of the drunk drivers involved in fatal accidents (Barakat and Mulinazzi 1987, 195; Doege and Engelberg 1986, 57). Their accidents are particularly associated with complex traffic situations, such as turning and joining vehicle streams in urban areas (Allgier 1965; Huston and Janke 1986). These are clearly situations in which late-age deficits – in recovery from glare, peripheral vision, dynamic visual acuity, and cognitive processing speeds – are a handicap to safe manoeuvring.

The relatively low period road accident and death rates among elderly drivers are partly explained by the benefits of experience, their avoidance of risk and their compensatory driving strategies and tactics. The interactive effects of age and experience was shown for London Transport bus drivers during the 1950s (Norman 1962, Table 13, citing Spratling 1961). All accidents, including minor shunts within the depots, were recorded and expressed as an annual rate per driver. At that time, drivers were employed to age 70 years. The accident rate was exceptionally low in drivers of all ages with at least 14 years experience, only rising modestly among the 60+ years (Figure 2.5). A stronger age relationship was present after 65 years among less experienced drivers. The most accident prone were aged less than 30 years with little experience.

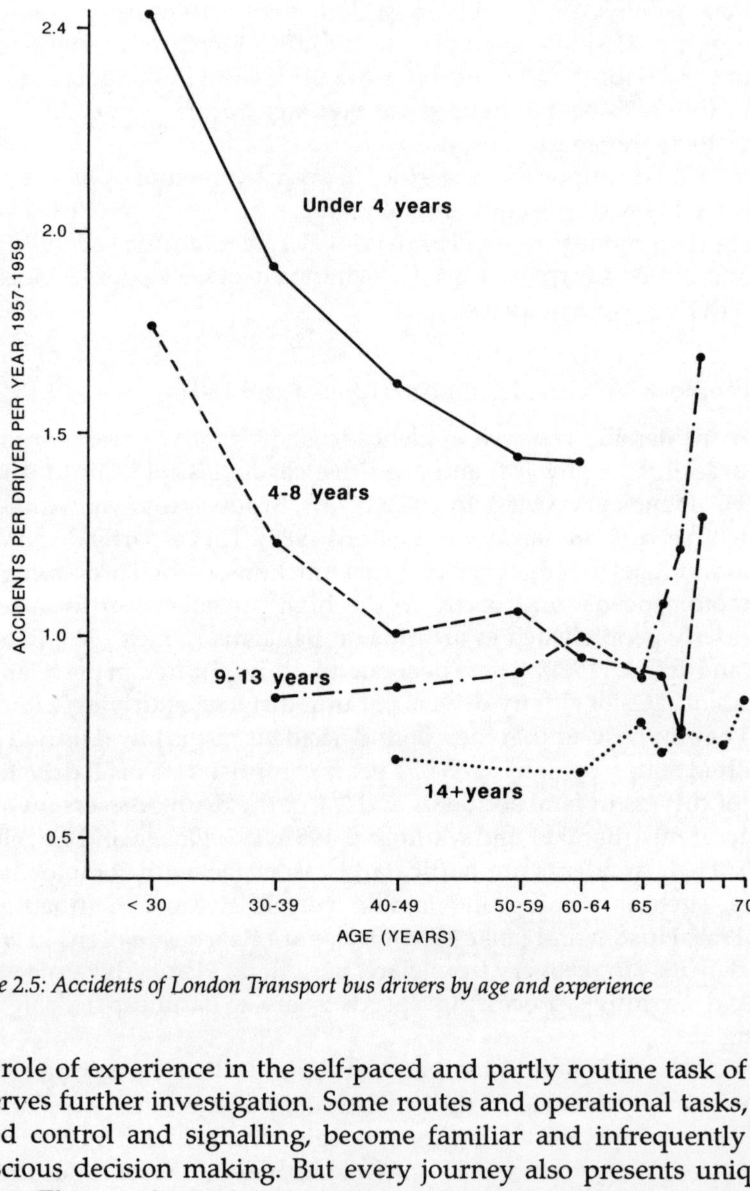

Figure 2.5: Accidents of London Transport bus drivers by age and experience

The role of experience in the self-paced and partly routine task of driving deserves further investigation. Some routes and operational tasks, such as speed control and signalling, become familiar and infrequently require conscious decision making. But every journey also presents unique situations. There is limited knowledge of the traffic situations which most expose the decreased physiological and cognitive abilities of older drivers. Recent experimental research on age-experience interactions have examined relatively simple operations, like typing, or abstract and generic cognitive tasks (Salthouse 1987, 1990). It is tempting to interpolate the experimental findings (which show experience to be a stronger influence on performance than age) from simpler tasks to driving. Driving's heavy load of sensory inputs, multiple task performance, and intermittently high information processing requirements indicate, however, differences of kind and not just degree. Age-related decrements in performance are known to be more severe in multiple than single cognitive tasks (Rabbitt 1977; van Wolffelaar and Rothengatter 1990). More understanding is certainly required, and this will involve difficult extensions of experimental research from readily defined and measured to complex multidimensional tasks.

The compensatory strategies and tactics adopted by elderly drivers are well described at the strategic, tactical and operational levels (Michon 1989; van Wolffelaar, Rothengatter and Brouwer 1987). All surveys find a significant proportion of elderly drivers refusing to drive at night, in bad weather conditions, on long journeys, at rush hours, through busy junctions or on unlit or unfamiliar roads (AA Foundation for Road Safety Research 1988). Stratagems include making journeys at quiet times of the day or on less busy minor roads and, in extreme cases, avoiding all turns across traffic flows. Tactics which consciously or unconsciously compensate for reduced physical and cognitive abilities include slower speeds, high vehicle separation distances (leading in merging manoeuvres to a common source of delay), greater lateral clearances, more frequent rests on long journeys and banning conversation or other distractions while driving. Compensatory behaviour can rarely be implemented in responsive driving operations of tracking and speed control. Unexpected vehicle and pedestrian movements cause particular problems.

Elderly road users are in fact most vulnerable as pedestrians. In many countries they account for more than one-fifth of pedestrian fatalities. This high accident rate is a consequence of their reduced physical, visual and cognitive abilities and a poor ability to anticipate traffic and vehicle behaviour (Sheppard and Pattinson 1986). The last disadvantage may in the present generation be linked to the absence of driving experience.

New Technology and the Older Driver

Elderly drivers take a responsible approach to their use of cars, readily admit at least some of their reduced competences, and are conscious of some of their own risk-avoidance strategies (Sixsmith, Rough and Warnes 1990). Ignorance of critical deficiencies and a reluctance to admit them can also be recognised. Visual decrements are more readily admitted than cognitive deficiencies. Many elderly drivers perceive their driving problems as caused by the inconsiderate, aggressive and illegal driving of young people.

The risk-avoidance and compensatory behaviours which have been described are self-actuated but rarely informed by measured evidence about a person's driving skills. There may be both safety and personal mobility benefits to experienced drivers of all ages from objective evaluation followed by specific training. There is little experience of such counselling except for drivers following severe accident traumas. Elderly drivers are receptive to information technologies involving new traffic or routing information devices designed to assist the driver (Sixsmith, Rough and Warnes 1990). While the theoretical possibility can be recognised of designing systems to help drivers identify their reduced competences and inappropriate driving styles, only recently have systematic attempts been made to understand how best to train people to drive safely. 'Driving is a self-paced task, in which drivers meet personal criteria of safety by attempting to match perceived habits in traffic to their perceived abilities to cope with those hazards' (Brown 1989). We need to know much more about how people internalise their knowledge of their skills and relate these to their own approach to driving.

During the last few years, the Commission of the European Communities, the United States Federal Highway Administration and the Japanese government have all initiated research programmes to investigate the potential of new information technology devices and systems for improving the capacity, efficiency and safety of vehicles and road networks. These may have particular value for older drivers. The CEC DRIVE Research Programme involves over 60 projects examining such technologies as integrated traffic management, route guidance systems, road pricing and automated vehicle control (Commission of the European Communities 1990). In the USA, researchers are concentrating on three technologies: computerised dashboard maps as route guidance, interactive traffic management systems based on roadside sensors, and speed and braking control systems for collision avoidance and to restrain illegal speeds (New York Times, 12 April, 1990).

With respect to elderly drivers, the theoretical advantages are clear. All drivers have a finite period capacity for receiving and acting upon information and this leads to errors and accidents in stress situations. Elderly drivers have lower capacities than younger drivers, putting them at a particular disadvantage. It could be beneficial either to take some processing tasks away from drivers, or to redistribute the tasks in time. For example, if a driver is informed in advance which road to take at a junction, one source of distraction is removed. On unfamiliar journeys, a route guidance system could inform the driver of the turn and traffic lane required before a junction is reached. The design and engineering of such systems raises, however, a host of problems. Whenever information is given to a driver, it inevitably distracts from other tasks. Much more needs to be known about the consequences of presenting additional information in different modes and at system or driver determined times.

The development of improved vehicle and highway safety measures including information devices for older drivers (and others with below average driving skills) could simultaneously serve traffic safety, motor industry, personal independence and morale, and social welfare goals. New information technology devices may be particularly valuable in:

(a) identifying the shortcomings of older people's driving skills and improving the accuracy of their self-assessments;

(b) providing information to drivers of reduced capacities which enables them to avoid more complex and stressful traffic situations, congested periods and difficult intersections and routes;

(c) providing a low cost and acceptable approach to retraining and tutoring; and

(d) providing a low cost approach to monitoring driving skills and identifying drivers who cannot raise their skills to acceptably safe standards.

Safety and Mobility Issues: Striking a Balance

The widening of inequalities in personal mobility between car users and others is a likely consequence of the spread of car use among the elderly population in both North America and Europe. As car ownership increases, on the one hand road investment climbs and new car-oriented shopping and leisure facilities are developed, while on the other, public transport usage declines, bus services are withdrawn, and the range and quality of city centre services decreases. These trends are reinforced by the redistribution of the population from high-density nucleated towns into far flung suburbs and fringe rural settlements. Elderly people, like all age groups, are becoming more dependent upon the private car for their mobility. The problem is that the more we adapt the road system and urban facilities for the growing number of drivers (including the affluent young retired), the more we are likely to compromise transport services for the non-driving, low income and single elderly population. Even taxi use and provision is declining in the United States. As public transport falls away, carless individuals will inevitably become more dependent on their friends, relatives and neighbours or on special community transport. But this last option is very expensive. In 1983 in the United States, community transport exclusive to elderly people cost $5.14 for a one-way trip. To provide special transportation services for all unlicensed elderly people so that they make as many trips as those with cars would cost $1.75 trillion annually (CSIMSOP 1988, 32).

The paradoxes for transport policy and investment of greater car dependency among the retired population extend from national policies to the standards for road and pavement design. Many 'improvements' to street furniture and layouts designed for safety reasons or to improve traffic flow, particularly the segregation of pedestrian movement with subways or bridges, increase the barriers and impediments to pedestrian movement. The assessment and notification of incompetent drivers engages general practitioners and psychogeriatricians in the resolution of an individual's independent mobility and their own safety, and in making judgements about the interests of the individual and of other road users.

In the public and professional spheres, more extensive car use among elderly people calls for supportive regulations and attitudes in fields unused to considering the circumstances of elderly people. Just as ageist attitudes survive in the health services and social administration, it is not surprising that they are commonplace among highway engineers and the motor industry. Personal transport and travel are regulated locally by the police and county or district highway departments and nationally by the Department of Transport. In these agencies, attitudes towards elderly drivers are sometimes disgracefully prejudiced. Legislation has been proposed in Florida to introduce an upper age limit of 80 years to hold a driving licence. More constructive attitudes will slowly prevail. It is encouraging that the transport professions have themselves become increasingly aware of the impacts of the ageing of the driving population. If some highway planners and regulators and motor engineers are initially anti-elderly, such attitudes arise from ignorance and the novelty of considering elderly people as a major road-user group.

References

Allgier, E. (1965) Accident involvements of older drivers. *Traffic Digest and Review* 13, 17–19.

Automobile Association Foundation for Road Safety Research (1988) *Motoring and the Older Driver,* Basingstoke, Hampshire: Automobile Association.

Barakat, S.J. and Mulinazzi, T.E. (1987) Elderly drivers: problems and needs for research. *Transportation Quarterly* 41 (2) 189–206.

Brown, I.D. (1989) *How Can We Train Safe Driving?* Groningen, Netherlands: Verkeerskundig Studiecentrum Rijksuniversiteit Groningen.

California Department of Motor Vehicles (1982) *Senior Driver Facts,* Sacramento, California: California Department of Motor Vehicles.

Carp, F.M. (1972) Transportation and retirement. *Proceedings of the American Society of Civil Engineers* TE4, 787–798.

Commission of the European Communities (1990) *DRIVE 90: The DRIVE Programme in 1990,* Brussels: Directorate General XIII, CEC.

Daniels, P.W. and Warnes, A.M. (1980) *Movement in Cities.* London: Methuen.

Department of Transport (1976) *Transport Statistics 1974/75.* London: HMSO.

Department of Transport (1988) *National Travel Survey 1985/86: Part 1: An Analysis of Personal Travel.* London: HMSO.

Department of Transport (1990) *Transport Statistics 1988/89.* London: HMSO.

Doege, T.C. and Engelberg, A.L. (eds) (1986) *Medical Conditions Affecting Drivers.* Chicago: American Medical Association.

Eisenhandler, S.A. (1990) The asphalt identikit: old age and the driver's licence. *International Journal of Aging and Human Development 30* (1) 1–14.

Florida Department of Highway Safety and Motor Vehicles (1990) *Driving Licences Issued in Florida,* Talahassee, Florida.

Graca, J.L. (1986) Driving and aging. *Clinical Geriatric Medicine 2,* 577–589.

Hagerstrand, T. (1967) *Innovation Diffusion as a Spatial Process.* Chicago: University of Chicago Press.

Hillman, M., Henderson, I. and Whalley, A. (1976) *Transport Realities and Planning Policy: Studies of Friction and Freedom in Daily Travel,* Report 42, London: Political and Economic Planning.

Huston, R. and Janke, M. (1986) *Senior Driver Facts,* Report 82. Sacramento: California Department of Motor Vehicles.

Kline, D.W. (1987) Ageing and human factors in transportation. *US National Research Council Workshop on Human Factors Research Issues for an Aging Population,* August 12–13, Washington D.C..

Markovitz, J.K. (1971) Transportation needs of the elderly. *Traffic Quarterly* 25, 237–53.

Michon, J.A. (1989) Explanatory pitfalls and rule-based driver models. *Accident Analysis and Prevention 21,* 341–353.

Norman, A. (1977) *Transport and the Elderly,* London: National Corporation for the Care of Old People.

Norman, L.G. (1962) *Road Traffic Accidents Epidemiology, Control and Prevention.* Geneva: World Health Organisation.

Office of Population Censuses and Surveys (1983) *Census of Great Britain 1981: Households and Household Composition*. London: HMSO.

Organisation for Economic Cooperation and Development (1985) *Traffic Safety of Elderly Road Users,* OECD, Paris.

Planek, T.W. and Overend, R. (1973) Profile of the aging driver. *Traffic Safety 73,* 37–39.

Ponds, R.W.H.M., Brouwer, W.H., and van Wolffelaar, P.C. (1988) Age differences in divided attention in a simulated driving task. *Journal of Gerontology 43,* 151–156.

Rabbitt, P.M.A. (1977) Changes in problem solving ability in old age. In J.E. Birren and K.W. Schaie (eds), *Handbook of the Psychology of Aging.* New York: Van Nostrand Reinhold, 913–919.

Retchin, S.M., Cox, J., Fox, M. and Irwin, L. (1988) Performance based measurements among elderly drivers and non-drivers. *Journal of the American Geriatrics Society 36,* 813–819.

Reuben, D.B., Silliman, R.A. and Traines, M. (1988) The aging driver: medicine, policy and ethics. *Journal of the American Geriatrics Society 36,* 1135–1142.

Robson, P. (1982) Patterns of activity and mobility among elderly people. In A.M. Warnes (ed.), *Geographical Perspectives on the Elderly,* Chichester: Wiley, 265–280.

Rogers, E.M. (1983) *The Diffusion of Innovations.* New York: Free Press.

Salthouse, T.A. (1987) Age, experience and compensation. In C. Schooler and K.W. Schaie (eds), *Cognitive Functioning and Social Structure over the Life Course.* Norwood, New Jersey: Ablex, 142–158.

Salthouse, T.A. (1990) Cognitive competence and expertise in aging. In J.E. Birren and K.W. Schaie (eds), *Handbook of the Psychology of Aging 3rd edtn,* New York: Academic, 310–319.

Sheppard, D. and Pattinson, I.M. (1986) *Interviews with Elderly Pedestrians Involved in Road Accidents.* Crowthorne, Berkshire: Research Report 88, Transport and Road Research Laboratory.

Sixsmith, J., Rough, B. and Warnes, A.M. (1990) Elderly Drivers Attitudes to RTI Devices: A Report of Group Discussions, *EC DRIVE Programme, Project V1006 'DRIVAGE', Deliverable 3,* Department of Geography, King's College, London.

Spratling, F.H. (1961) *British Transport Review 6,* 172.

Taira, E.D. (1989) *Assessing the Driving Ability of the Elderly: A Preliminary Investigation.*New York: Haworth.

Thomson, M. (1977) *Great Cities and Their Traffic,* London: Penguin.

USA Committee for the Study on Improving Mobility and Safety for Older Persons (CSIMSOP) (1988) *Transportation in an Aging Society: Improving Mobility and Safety for Older Persons, Volume 1, Committee Report and Recommendations,* Washington D.C.: Transportation Research Board, National Research Council.

van Wolffelaar, P., Rothengatter, T. and Brouwer, W. (1987) Compensation strategies of elderly car drivers. *Proceedings of the Ergonomics Society Annual Conference 1987,* London: Taylor & Francis, 95–100.

van Wolffelaar, P. and Rothengatter, T. (1990) Divided Attention in RTI-tasks for Elderly Drivers, *EC DRIVE Programme, Project V1006 'DRIVAGE', Deliverable 2,* Traffic Research Centre, University of Groningen.

Warnes, A.M. (1989) Factors in elderly people's driving abilities. *EC DRIVE Programme, Project V1006 'DRIVAGE', Deliverable 1,* Department of Geography, King's College, London.

Welford, A.T. (1982) Motor skills and aging. In J.A. Mortimer, F.J. Priozzolo and G.J. Maletta (eds), *The Aging Motor System.* New York: Praeger.

CHAPTER 3

Literacy and Older Adults

Alexandra Withnall

The arrival of International Literacy Year in 1990 – although seriously under-resourced in the United Kingdom – helped to focus attention on the nature and extent of problems caused by illiteracy in the developing nations. However, for the last two decades, there has been a growth in concern about the social and educational issues surrounding adult illiteracy in industrialised countries. In Britain, for example, these issues have been brought sharply into focus in recent times by the fierce debate in both the educational and popular press regarding the standards of attainment in reading, writing and numeracy achieved by school children and young people. In particular, this debate has focused on whether standards are declining or improving over time, and the likely consequences for the future of the economy of a workforce whose abilities in literacy are poor.

Limage (1990) has examined in depth the growth of recognition of the complex issues surrounding adult illiteracy in North America and in Western European countries. In particular, she discusses the need for awareness-raising as a first step in addressing adult literacy, the importance of a public commitment of resources, the development of partnerships to enable need to be identified and appropriate provision made and, perhaps most importantly, the argument that literacy is a basic human right, not something which can be justified purely in economic terms. This point was also stressed in the Declaration adopted by participants at the International Seminar on Literacy in Industrialized Countries held in Toronto in 1987 (Gayfer 1987).

In England and Wales, provision for adult literacy and associated basic skills is the responsibility of the Adult Literacy and Basic Skills Unit (ALBSU) which has its mandate and budget renewed on a rolling basis by the Department of Education and Science. As well as acting as the central focus for basic skills work with adults, ALBSU provides a consultancy and advisory service for Local Education Authorities (LEAs), voluntary bodies and other organisations, and sponsors a range of development projects, staff training and development, and allocates grants to voluntary organisations. It has also produced and published a wide range of teaching and learning materials and sponsors occasional research (ALBSU 1989a).

In spite of this activity, ALBSU is very much aware that current provision reaches only the tip of the iceberg of estimated need. In most areas of England

and Wales, the available service is barely able to cope. It appears that whilst the very best local education authority is providing for about 4% of the estimated number in need at any time, the poorest provider can only offer tuition to less than 0.05% of the estimated number of adults in need. 'The cost in social, economic and human terms of this gap between need and available provision is staggering' (ALBSU 1989b, p.5).

Although local education authorities are the major providers, in most areas there is increasing recognition, as has been seen, that a thorough mastery of literacy and numeracy is an essential pre-requisite for most vocational training and for the development of a competent workforce. Hence the impetus given to the acquisition of basic skills in programmes such as Employment Training and the Youth Training Scheme by the now defunct Training Agency and currently run under the auspices of the Training and Enterprise Councils (TECs). Adults also receive tuition in prisons and other penal establishments and through agencies such as the probation service, hospitals and adult training centres. Currently, ALBSU is undertaking a major initiative together with the BBC and other government departments to provide a system of accreditation for learning at four levels which will sit within the National Council for Vocational Qualifications framework (NCVQ).

It has been observed that the key factor in the development of the British adult literacy and basic skills experience appears to be its pragmatism in dealing with changing public awareness and expressed need as well as the precariousness of funding. Yet, in recent times, this pragmatism has been confronted by increased demand for financial accountability, especially at the local level as expressed in the controversy surrounding the 1988 Education Reform Act (Limage 1990). It is surely important that, in the current political and economic situation, we do not lose sight of the basic philosophy behind the provision of adult literacy tuition – literacy as a basic human right for the advancement of everyone in society, not just provision to be justified in economic terms.

Older People and Learning Activity

This philosophy takes on a particular importance in relation to the situation of the population of people over state retirement age. There has been very little discussion or research in Britain about how older people fare in a society which increasingly emphasises proficiency in a range of skills as a means not just for economic survival but also in order to acquire the understanding and ability to survive in a complex and fast moving world.

Changing demographic trends are now impinging on the public consciousness. In mid 1985, the estimated population aged over 60 years in Britain was 11.4 million – about 20% of the population – with women accounting for three out of every five persons. To the end of the century, it is expected that the number of people in their sixties will actually decline, but the number of people aged 80 and over will increase rapidly from 1.8 million in 1985 to 2.4 million in 2001, and 2.6 million in 2011 (Thompson 1987). Of course, this sector of the population is by no means homogenous in its make-up; we can reasonably assume, however, that many people now retired received limited schooling in the past. Almost all certainly experienced some degree of disruption to their lives during the Second World War. It appears, as shown by available statistical evidence, that they do not avail themselves of opportunities for formal learning activity in retirement to any great degree. Neither is any information available as to their participation in literacy activities, although individual accounts have been collected by Age Concern's Forum on the Rights of Elderly People to Education (FREE 1990). Because of these factors, they are often further disadvantaged by the widely held belief that minimal formal schooling and lack of educational qualifications must be automatically equated with dependency and poor quality of life in the later years. Such a perspective ignores the fact that, of course, many older people are involved in a range of activities in clubs, societies, churches, voluntary organisations or with family responsibilities for grandchildren or other relatives. Percy (1990a) has commented that, as yet, we do not know or understand the manner in which learning in non-formal settings arise organically out of the lives of the learners. If we can develop appropriate models and parameters of non-formal learning, we might then be able to investigate the levels of participation of older adults in this kind of learning and the subsequent outcomes for their lives.

Perspectives of Adult Literacy

Because of this lack of any firm evidence, it is not possible to state categorically that older people are less literate than any other sector of the population, or that they find literacy a problem in their lives. In the USA, where educators have tried to promote literacy programmes specifically for older adults, Kasworm and Medina (1989) have addressed the question by reviewing the literature on meanings of literacy; they categorise the major perspectives of adult literacy into four orientations of the concept for the learner in relation to a societal context.

1. Primary Life Skills State

This perspective focuses upon basic skills in the sense that it is used by ALBSU: 'skills for fundamental human symbolic interaction, living tasks and basic knowledge and skills for exchange between people and society' (p.67). These include reading, writing and oral communication, computational and problem-solving skills. We may want to add facility in English by those whose mother tongue is not English and computer literacy to the list – in other words, life-coping skills and skills to meet everyday needs. However, establishing accurate measures of basic skills abilities in order to decide at what point a person has acquired an adequate set of functional abilities at a particular time presents a complex problem (ALBSU 1987). It could be argued that few people, if any, really possess all the multiple skills required to function effectively in an advanced industrial society undergoing rapid social, economic and technological change. High levels of technical competence in, for example, reading, are no guarantee that these skills can be used and translated into action when required.

2. Normative Literacy Policy State

This is described as the enacted policy or assumed normative level of skills and knowledge for basic literacy in a particular cultural or environmental context. For example, different professional/organisational groupings may establish, through a policy decision, certain standards of entry to particular jobs or educational courses (in Britain, many employers require young people to have acquired General Certificate of Secondary Education (GCSE) passes in English Language and Mathematics as a minimum, and this is also mandatory for entry into various courses of professional training). Such a perspective is based upon educational achievement usually gained within a schooling context and is again related to notions of economic survival, a definition which may no longer be relevant for older people.

3. Culture-Bearer State

This perspective is based upon the assumption that an individual will not only be literate in the life skills described earlier, but will also be literate within what is called 'the culture of the educated' (p.68) and will be able to provide leadership to this culture and perhaps improve the condition and quality of life through his/her role. It is not a perspective which has been discussed in relation to adult literacy in Britain, but it does offer the possibility of further investigation as an issue in respect of older people. There are, after all, many examples within the fields of literature and the arts, of older people who provide respected leadership by virtue of their longevity and hence through their experience and achievement in their particular fields.

4. Self-sufficiency State

The implication here is that literacy is based in the person's concept of life roles and culture. It is defined as the skills and knowledge perceived by the individual to be necessary to his/her role as a responsible interacting adult operating within a particular environment and contributing, as an adult, to significant others. It is the ethos of the individual and his/her current life which provides the basis to define what literacy means and what is competent adult performance.

Viewed from this perspective, literacy can offer a sense of empowerment in the tradition of Freire's (1973) emphasis on making people critically conscious of their condition and helping them eliminate oppressive factors in communal life. As yet, in Britain, we have not seen older people developing a political consciousness in respect of their apparently marginalised position in society to the same extent as, for example, in the USA where the Gray Panthers have appeared as a recognisable force. This may be because, as Percy (1990b) points out, there are difficulties in generalising about older people as a disadvantaged or disempowered group uniformly requiring both freedom and power. The heterogeneity of the older age group needs to be both recognised and respected.

From this overview of meanings ascribed to literacy, it appears that no one definition is strictly applicable to the situation of older people in Britain. However, it does seem doubtful that literacy and associated basic skills can be categorised merely as a discrete set of useful tools which can be acquired at an early stage and then put to use as an when required throughout the lifespan.

A more attractive definition is that of competencies which an individual perceives as important in order to sustain his/her lifestyle at a particular point. There may be activities or demands which acquire significance at particular ages for different people and which require the rapid development of a certain skill or body of knowledge for a specific purpose. It might be assumed that retirement is a particular phase of the lifecourse which makes such new demands on the individual as well as offering fresh opportunities for personal development.

Researching Older People's Use of Literacy

Because of the lack of empirical research in Britain surrounding this issue, a pilot study was set up to examine: (i) what literacy skills (using the 'basic skills' definition, i.e. reading, writing, oral communication and computational activities) a small sample of adults actually use in their daily lives during retirement; (ii) whether they seek assistance with basic skills and from whom; and (iii) what aspects of their abilities in basic skills they would wish to improve, if any. In addition, it was hoped that the pilot study might also have implications for the methodology of researching aspects of old age.

The focus of the pilot study was a West Midlands metropolitan borough where the 1981 Census reported the population of pensionable age and over as 15.6% of the usually resident population (men = 5.1%, women = 10.6%). At that time 4.6% of the population were then aged 75 years and over. Calculations from more recent Office of Population Censuses and Surveys (OPCS) data suggest that this older age group is increasing in its numbers. In 1989, when the pilot study was carried out, the borough's Mayor inaugurated an Age Awareness Campaign to focus attention on the area's senior citizens both to help improve their lives practically and socially and to increase awareness of ageing issues among younger age groups.

Retired people are catered for in the borough through a comprehensive range of services including free access to learning opportunities in educational establishments and community centres as well as through leisure and recreational activities, library and museum services and a number of senior citizens groups including the University of the Third Age. (The British University of the Third Age, formally constituted in 1984, is a loose federation of self-help groups of older people practising a variety of learning/studying processes ranging from traditional but unpaid teaching to learning exchanges. No qualifications are required and there are no distinctions between teachers and students.) There is also a flourishing LEA-funded adult basic education scheme with a full-time organiser offering provision throughout the borough. However, take-up of formal learning opportunities among older people is apparently low.

The initial problem to be faced was that of gaining access to a sample of retired people who would be willing to be interviewed. Particular sensitivity is required when asking questions about abilities in, and use of basic skills, since people obviously do not want to be seen in some way 'deficient' in the eyes of others. Initially, possible respondents were approached through church-based social clubs for retired people. However, the general unwillingness to participate in the pilot study which emerged was apparently not related to the subject of the study but to the fact that potential respondents had recently been in receipt of Community Charge/Poll Tax registration forms and exhibited considerable alarm at being approached by interviewers whom they saw as in some way connected with officialdom and bureaucracy. Older people's very real fears about official intrusion into their privacy and issues of confidentiality obviously need to be taken into account if they are to be asked to participate in qualitative research. The timing of any fieldwork also requires consideration.

Data were eventually gathered by a trained interviewer who was able to identify a small random sample of retired people living in two electoral wards in the north of the borough. This interviewer had already made contact with respondents as part of a larger market research project which had involved a house-to-house survey of people over 60 years of age in that area. As a result, she was already known to and trusted by respondents, was welcomed into their homes and was confident in her ability to elicit the required information with sensitivity and to judge the validity of responses. Although it is not claimed that the method of selecting respondents described above provides a representative sample of all elderly people, it afforded access to a pilot study population and the results obtained gave indications of questions which would need to be investigated in any larger scale survey.

Summary of Findings

1. Characteristics of respondents

A total of 20 people were interviewed. Five were aged 60–64, eight were in the 65–69 age bracket and the other seven were aged 70 plus. The youngest respondent was a women of 60 and the oldest a widower of 91. Clearly, these two respondents were a generation apart in age and likely to have had quite different life experiences. Apart from the widower, one man was single whilst the other men were all married; of the women, eight were widowed and the remainder married. Among the widows, four were in the older age group, but the others were still in their sixties. Ten respondents lived with a spouse and six completely alone; one lived with an adult son and three with other relations. In spite of these differing situations, all the respondents were reasonably fit and led independent lives. Nine felt they had no particular health problems which in any way impaired their physical abilities. Three others wore glasses and had hearing aids fitted whilst eight others used glasses for reading only.

Some attempt was made to learn about respondents' backgrounds by asking their age on leaving school and obtaining details of their last occupation prior to retirement. Seventeen of the sample had left school at 14, one at 16 and the other two equated 'school' with 'formal education' since further questioning revealed that both had subsequently trained as teachers on leaving school. They described 'school' as continuing into their twenties. Although there is no firm evidence as to whether age is a reliable guide to people's response capacities, interviewers need to be aware of possible age-related variations in vocabulary usage and in verbal fluency (Withnall 1989).

Respondents had worked in a wide variety of occupations although one woman had never been in paid employment. Apart from the two teachers, most had ended their working lives in unskilled or semi-skilled occupations with clerical work and jobs in the leather trade – for which the borough is noted – featuring predominantly. Respondents were not asked what skills they had used in their employment, but a more sophisticated survey of basic skills usage could be developed to elicit this information in the future.

What was perhaps more pertinent to the survey was the description respondents gave of their activities in retirement. Only three currently attended any form of adult education class, one of these being provided by a trade union for its retired members, one by a retirement council and the other by the LEA. Although eight had no formal membership of any organisation, two belonged to – and were apparently active in – a pensioners' political action group; in addition, five belonged to a church organisation; three to a golf club, and two regularly attended a Senior Citizen's Group. Only one women perceived that her activities – within a Sunday School – involved her in additional reading and writing activity. However, respondents had developed a very wide range of hobbies and interests, usually a continuation of an interest they had enjoyed prior to retirement.

Hobbies included knitting, music, reading, DIY, carpentry, organ-playing, growing bonsai trees, golf, dancing, gardening, marquetry, sewing, bingo and generally watching television. Presumably, these activities must require participants to have acquired a sound grasp of basic skills and to be able to apply them in some quite complex situations. Even a 'passive' hobby such as watching television involves the viewer in reading programme schedules in order to make a decision as to what shall be viewed on a particular day.

2. *Reading*

Only one respondent, a married woman in the older age group, stated absolutely that she did not enjoy reading. The interviewer asked respondents whether they read a wide selection of materials such as newspapers/magazines, books, dictionaries/reference books, instructions, official forms, circulars/advertisements and letters on a regular basis and whether they did each of these easily or with difficulty. They were also asked if there were any aspects of their reading abilities which they would like to improve. Of course, there are inherent methodological difficulties in asking for self-reported accounts of activity in reading since people's perceptions of their abilities may not accord with objective reality. There also still exists the stigma of 'illiteracy' which many people would be at pains to conceal. However, since interest was primarily in the way in which older people use basic skills within their own life contexts, these perceptions were of prime importance.

Only five of the respondents stated that they had occasion to read all the items listed on a regular basis – although of course it is not clear what meaning this phrase has for the individual without a more closely structured interview schedule. Nineteen of the sample read newspapers and magazines and 16 read fiction/non-fiction and letters easily. Least consulted were dictionaries and reference books, and circulars/advertisements were largely ignored.

Two people admitted difficulties in reading instructions and official forms; two also added: 'My husband/wife deals with the forms'. Only one respondent reported difficulty in reading a newspaper: 'I can't concentrate on rubbish'.

One man gave examples of his current reading interests – a history of the First World War and a regular periodical, *Know Your Plants*. One woman felt that she would like to improve her reading abilities in order to be able to understand 'historical books' and learn a foreign language properly. The other respondents did not see any necessity to improve any aspect of their reading abilities.

Subjects were asked who they turn to first when they encounter a difficulty with written material. Two of the married women, perhaps surprisingly, would not consult anyone; three respondents identified an official at the Civic Centre or Neighbourhood Office as a source of help, but the remainder would rely on relatives for assistance. However, a typical comment was: 'I don't usually have any difficulties'.

In future, it might be more appropriate to develop a reading inventory designed to define reading habits in more detail (Scales and Biggs 1987), or to develop the survey to include questions relating to how respondents had learnt to read, their perceptions of their general reading ability, how much time they spent reading and whether they felt their abilities had improved or declined over the years (Heisel and Larson 1984).

3. Writing

Nine of the sample commented that they did not enjoy writing, although the interviewer did not distinguish between handwriting and 'functional' writing. Three of these avoided any writing tasks whatsoever. However, 16 of the sample found it necessary to deal with official forms from time to time, 13 wrote regular letters to friends and relatives and 11 of these were also able to construct a formal letter to an official body. Nine people enjoyed crossword puzzles / word games and competitions although, as was noted in the previous section, they did not make as much use of dictionaries and reference books to assist them as might have been expected.

Respondents identified more difficulties with writing tasks than with reading. Four people admitted to difficulties with filling in official forms: 'Sometimes you don't understand what they mean'. The same respondent added, 'I suppose I could fill forms up, but I always leave them to my sons'.

The three people who avoided any writing tasks apparently relied on a spouse to deal with official forms. Asked whether there was anything connected with writing which they would like to be better at, two respondents mentioned spelling and one handwriting: 'I'd like to do better writing. I'd like to have one particular style'. However, the general view was that it was too late to improve: 'Not really now, but I wish I had been better in the past'.

For assistance with any task involving writing, 17 of the sample would once again turn to relatives and one to an official at the Civic Centre. The two people who would not seek assistance with reading difficulties were prepared to ask relatives for help with writing whilst two other people would not seek help at all.

In future, it would be more appropriate to draw a distinction, when developing an interview schedule, between handwriting itself and actual use of writing as a medium of communication. Almost half the sample enjoyed the challenge of activities such as puzzles and competitions which require little ability in handwriting. It may be that older people's dislike of writing activity, where this was noted, is connected with physical impairment, such as poor eyesight, difficulties in holding a pen, forming letters, and so on as with being unable to respond adequately to 'forms'; difficulties of which older people themselves may be unaware.

4. Oral communication (talking and listening)

There are inherent difficulties in questioning anyone, whatever their age, about skills in oral communication since, if their skills are poor, they may not be able to describe what it is they find difficult. However, those who work in, for example, reminiscence are well aware that older people often have highly developed skills of recall and of story-telling. The interviewer, when asking about possible difficulties in understanding other people, used examples of situations such as telephone, television, chatting with friends, talking to people in shops, communicating with officials, and doctor's visits as prompts. Respondents were also asked whether they ever had difficulties making themselves understood. Two people sometimes had trouble understanding others due to hearing problems; but the oldest man in the survey commented: 'I wish people would stop asking me whether I want them to repeat what they've said'.

Four people admitted they sometimes had difficulties in explaining themselves to others, but were unable to describe the nature of their difficulties. Four other people described aspects of their spoken English which they would like to improve, mostly relating to a desire to become more articulate and improve their speech by ridding themselves of their very pronounced local accents. However, they were resigned to the fact that this was unlikely: 'I'll never alter now, will I?'

Older people's use of oral communication skills might be the subject of a separate, in-depth study in which respondents are asked how they respond to a range of situations relating to aspects of communication such as seeking information, holding long conversations at various levels including giving opinions and understanding argument, reactions to TV and radio programmes, conversing with children and so on. Such research would also need to take into account any possible conventions about what topics may be discussed aloud and how they can be discussed (see Ford and Sinclair 1987).

Allowance would have to be made for any age-related physical impairments which respondents might perceive as causing them particular difficulties.

5. Computation

Respondents were told that these final questions related to 'the sort of maths they used in every day life' and how they got on. Interestingly, use of the word 'maths' (for which the interviewer substituted 'numbers' at a later point) led to the kind of 'panic' in some respondents which Buxton (1981) has described as a pathological terror of mathematics often induced by memories of fear and embarrassment from past learning experiences rather than actual mental incapacity. Several respondents recalled in detail how strict discipline had been at school, terrors of mental arithmetic and being required to give quick responses, being tested by the Chairman of the Governors unexpectedly, fear of the cane and of being made to look silly in front of others. The interviewer had to exercise considerable tact and skill in reassuring some respondents that she was not intending to 'test' them in any way.

In fact, respondents were asked, first, about their activities involving financial transactions and how easy they found it to cope. Examples were understanding pensions and Department of Social Security (DSS) payments, reading bank/building society statements, checking bills, working out credit payments, and so on. Subjects were reasonably confident in dealing with these, although two people reported some difficulty understanding DSS payments. Although no questions were formally asked about the forthcoming Community Charge/Poll Tax, almost half the respondents tried to engage the interviewer in discussion about the implications of this for older people and exhibited considerable disquiet over whether they would understand how their contribution was to be calculated and what they would be expected to pay. (This new form of local taxation was introduced in England and Wales in 1990 and involved a completion by everyone over the age of 18 of detailed registration forms. It is to be replaced, following considerable public opposition, by a different form of local taxation in 1993.)

Regarding more practical applications of numeracy, three respondents complained of difficulties in estimating – for example, quantities such as paint and wallpaper, carpet areas or using the twenty-four-hour clock to set times for central heating and hot water. However, the major problem for eight respondents was the use of metric measurement for practical activities such as cooking or woodwork. Typical comments were, 'I've no clue about these new measurements. I don't think many of us have at our age'. 'I can work out weights better in the old way'. 'I can't do this metric system. I was brought up on the old system. I don't think people of my age can do metric'.

In spite of their unhappy earlier experiences, respondents reported themselves generally able to cope with arithmetical procedures such as addition, subtraction, multiplication, division, decimals and percentages, although they did not always recognise the mathematical symbol for each activity. One woman admitted to difficulties regarding multiplication and division and both she and another female respondent had problems with decimals and percentages. It may be asked to what extent respondents actually unconsciously performed calculations and used arithmetical techniques in their daily lives, especially in conjunction with hobbies, some of which appear to require an advanced facility in manipulating numbers and estimating quantities.

Respondents were shown a scientific calculator and asked if they knew how to use one. Perhaps surprisingly, only two respondents, both women, stated they definitely did not; the remaining respondents either already could use a calculator or qualified their answer: 'Yes, I'm sure I could if I was shown'.

To what extent do these very positive responses reflect reality and to what extent do they demonstrate that older people, when faced with modern technology, do not wish to seem old-fashioned or 'out-of-touch'? Certainly, there have been instances reported of older people gaining enormous satisfaction from learning computer skills. There is no prima facie reason why previous difficulties with numerical concepts should now prevent older people from taking advantage of technological development to further their skill development in the same way as their grand-children take these skills for granted.

On the whole, respondents were not concerned to improve their mathematical abilities except for one women who cited decimals as an area where she was 'never any good at school'. Fourteen people turned to relatives once again for help with anything connected with numerical skills, although one person would prefer not to seek any assistance. The other respondents said they would be more likely to turn to someone at the Neighbourhood Office or Civic Centre for help in dealing with numeracy problems. This may reflect society's apparent belief that to be – and to admit to being – innumerate is in some way more acceptable than being illiterate.

Bearing in mind these respondents' fearful reactions to questions regarding numerical and mathematical usage, a further study might utilise a different research strategy. For example, a more revealing way of examining what concepts they need to use in daily life might be to ask a cross-section of older people in a particular area to keep a diary for a short period of time noting down what kinds of calculations they used in what situations and when they needed to seek help. Such a study might reveal whether people in different phases of retirement need to acquire particular numerical skills at any point; and whether women who generally have responsibility for the day-to-day running of a household utilise practical mathematics to a greater extent than they realised. At the time of the survey, it was apparent that understanding the practical financial implications of the Community Charge was looming as an important issue in the lives of respondents; how they learn about this might also provide the basis for further study.

Research and the Educational Needs of Older Adults

If we accept the validity of the foregoing responses, it appears that most of the older people interviewed were meeting their self-defined needs in the area of basic skills as categorised here. They did not appear to see themselves as in any way 'excluded' from participation in society although they were often aware of deficiencies in some aspects of their abilities. Nevertheless, if they did encounter problems, they could turn to a relative or knew where to seek help and advice. Wenger, in her analysis of the support networks used by elderly people, has commented that they may have access to different sorts of support within a community; the older people in our survey appeared to belong to what she has categorised as a local integrated support network of family and close relatives, often based on long-established residence (Wenger 1989).

In the USA, Fingeret (1983) has commented that people with specific literacy needs often belong to a social network of family and friends through which they obtain help with reading and writing difficulties in exchange for giving other kinds of help. She argues that such interaction is based on the concept of reciprocity and in no way involves dependence on the part of those seeking help with basic skills. Nor does any social stigma attach to them. Her findings seem to confirm the notion that access to skills and information may indeed be as important as possession (Fingeret 1983). How far respondents were involved in providing other kinds of help to relatives who assisted them with basic skills was not investigated at this stage, but this aspect of the helping relationship does merit further exploration and analysis.

There appeared to be little interest among respondents in improving basic skills except in a few instances. It may be that they needed more time to assess in which areas they would like to acquire skills than the researcher was able to give. However, ALBSU's experience is that older people do not seek help from adult basic education schemes in any great numbers. It seems unlikely, therefore, that basic education schemes, such as literacy programmes in the USA under the auspices of the National Council on Aging, would meet with much success in this country. A more appropriate response might be, as Fingeret advocates, to offer training, support and materials to those in network contact with people (of all ages) who have to seek help with aspects of basic skills usage. However, considerable prior groundwork would be required to identify the networks and reciprocities involved, the nature of the training required and the contexts in which it could be provided.

The respondents in the pilot study were generally physically fit, able to get about easily and living with, or within reach of immediate family members. It cannot be said with any certainty that other older people living within what Wenger (1989) terms a private restricted support network – characterised by absence of local kin or friends and perhaps having only superficial contact with neighbours and limited knowledge of the local community – would be able to cope with the basic skill requirements of their daily lives in the same way as these respondents. The predicted increase in the numbers of very old people in the population towards the close of the century was noted earlier. Further research is required here to illuminate how older adults use and gain access to basic skills and knowledge within their individual social contexts in the later phases of retirement when they may have no immediate relatives or contacts with whom to establish a reciprocal relationship.

The Needs of Ethnic Minorities

The situation of the elders in ethnic minority groups also merits consideration. In a recent study of the need for English for speakers of other languages, 44% of those questioned in the 56+ age group lacked proficiency in understanding, speaking, reading and writing English (ALBSU 1989c). At present, we do not know how older members of the ethnic minority groups fare in a society which emphasises proficiency in English language and familiarity with a particular numerical system as the main source of knowledge, power and culture. Nor do we have any understanding of whether older members of different language groups are motivated to improve their abilities in basic skills including learning English. For members of ethnic minorities who have also poorly developed skills in their mother tongue, problems of dependency are likely to be compounded. However, the issues involved in the processes of becoming and being literate are complex. Ferdman (1990) has argued that in a multi-ethnic society, literacy is culturally framed and defined and that members of different cultures will obviously vary in what they perceive as literate behaviour. This in turn can influence how individuals engage in literacy acquisition and activity. In addition, the type and content of literacy education that individuals receive can also influence their cultural identity. The connections between literacy and culture need to be acknowledged and more fully understood in order that literacy can become a universal characteristic of society.

The arguments for literacy as a tool for empowering the learner have already been examined. Certainly, many gerontologists may wish to argue that, in spite of their heterogeneity, it will be increasingly important for older people through sheer weight of numbers to become aware of, and be able to use, the skills of self-advocacy in order to make policy-makers, the media and the public at large aware of the hitherto marginalised position of older people in society and the importance of issues which affect all older people and, ultimately, everyone. In this sense, literacy can aid older people to fulfil what Laslett (1989) calls 'their forward-reaching social responsibilities' and help them towards developing a political consciousness in respect of themselves and of succeeding generations. How far the responsibility for such empowerment should lie with the adult literacy tutor and to what extent he/she could actually begin to achieve this are, of course, debatable points.

Percy (1990a), in a critique of the 'empowerment' model of educational gerontology, proposes 'the notion of older people as teachers, facilitators of learning, role models, educational resources, repositories of wisdom…' (237). Certainly, there are examples in Britain of older people taking an active role in inter-generational learning programmes such as those run under the auspices of Help the Aged and Community Service Volunteers. In the USA, the concept of family literacy and inter-generational literacy programmes has been seen as one way to facilitate adaptation to changing demographies and lifestyles (Nickse 1990). There are many different examples of the genre currently operating in the USA, most of which appear to utilise a parent-child approach although other models exist. Their development has been accelerated by the need to support immigrant and refugee families' participation in their children's education. In this country, basic skills work with parents has been designated a priority by ALBSU and a number of development projects to test out different models are currently operational.

Experience from the USA suggests that such an approach is not without problems. Auerbach (1989) in a critical analysis of family literacy programmes which function under what she terms a new version of the 'deficit hypothesis', proposes a broader definition of family literacy which both acknowledges the family's social reality and focuses on the family's strengths. Hence, curriculum development would be informed by community concerns and cultural practices. Emergent issues could be explored and transformed into content-based literacy work so that literacy, in turn, also becomes a tool for shaping social context.

Nickse (1990) also warns of some of the challenges facing educators wishing to develop family/inter-generational literacy programmes. These include the complex planning and administrative procedures required, and the need for adequate funding, materials and accommodation. It appears also that family participation in planning can sometimes be a delicate process in that skills, behaviours and attitudes sometimes have to be changed leading to resentments and fears which are often difficult to confront. Sensitivity to cultural differences is also important, suggesting the need for intensive staff training in this kind of approach, especially as evaluation of success is likely to be a complex procedure.

If these difficulties can be acknowledged and accepted at the outset, such an approach offers the possibility of involving not just parents, but other family members, especially older people, in contributing to children's literacy development – and hence to their own learning and to their standing within the community. Truly inter-generational programmes could recruit older people who have no immediate family and capitalise on their skills and knowledge so that literacy for everyone becomes a community concern rather than a matter for individual shame. Alongside such developments must go longitudinal research to assess the effects of such activities in helping to break the cycle of illiteracy and in improving the quality of life for all participants.

Summary

As yet, there is very little research relating to older people and literacy in this country. However, it can be argued that literacy should not be defined externally as a clearly identifiable set of life coping skills, but must be based on an individual's self-perceived requirements within his/her own life context at any particular age. Although the pilot study of older people's use of literacy defined as basic skills was necessarily limited in its methodology and scope, its findings have raised a number of issues both for adult literacy and educational gerontology which have not previously been addressed.

Ironically, as awareness of demographic trends begins to impact on the employment market, there are signs that, in order to improve economic competitiveness, government and employers alike are coming to recognise that it will be necessary to encourage older people to stay on at work for a longer period or to re-enter employment and to widen access for older people to education and training opportunities. It may be that some of the issues relating to older people and literacy which have been raised here will necessarily come to assume a more critical importance during the 1990s as we move towards an ageless society. We need to identify and begin to understand these issues now.

References

Adult Literacy and Basic Skills Unit (1987) *Literacy, Numeracy and Adults, Evidence from the National Child Development Study, London.* Kingsbourne House, 229/231 High Holborn, London WC1V 7DA: ALBSU.

Adult Literacy and Basic Skills Unit (1989a) *Annual Report 1988–1989.* London: ALBSU.

Adult Literacy and Basic Skills Unit (1989b) *After the Act. Developing Basic Skills Work in the 1990s.* London: ALBSU.

Adult Literacy and Basic Skills Unit (1989c) *A Nation's Neglect: Research in to the Need for English Amongst Speakers of Other Languages.* London: ALBSU.

Auerbach, E.R. (1989) Towards a social – contextual approach to family literacy. *Harvard Education Review* 59 (2) 165–181.

Buxton, L. (1981) *Do You Panic About Maths?* London: Heinemann Educational.

Ferdman, B.M. (1990) Literacy and cultural identity. *Harvard Educational Review* 60 (2) 181–203.

Fingeret, A. (1983) Social networks: a new perspective on independence and illiterate adults. *Adult Education Quarterly* 33, 133–146.

Ford, J. and Sinclair, R. (1987) *Sixty Years On. Women Talk About Old Age*. London: The Women's Press.

Forum on the Rights of Elderly People to Education (1990) *FREE Newsletter* 38. Age Concern England, Bernard Sunley House, 60 Pitcairn Road, Mitcham, Surrey, CR4 3LL.

Freire, P. (1973) *Education for Critical Consciousness. London: Sheed and Ward.*

Gayfer, M. (ed) (1987) *Literacy in Industrialised Countries, A Focus on Practice.* Toronto: ICAE 29 Prince Arthur Avenue, Toronto, Canada, MSR 1B2.

Heisel, M. and Larson, G. (1984) Literacy and social milieu: reading behaviour of the black elderly. *Adult Education Quarterly* 34, 63–70.

Kasworm, C.E. and Medina, R.A. (1989) Perspectives of literacy in the senior adult years. *Educational Gerontology* 15, 65–79.

Laslett, P. (1989) *A Fresh Map of Life, The Emergence of the Third Age.* London: Weidenfeld and Nicholson.

Limage, L. (1990) Adult literacy and basic education in Europe and North America; from recognition to provision. *Comparative Education* 26 (1) 125–140.

Nickse, R. (1990) Family literacy and community education: prospects for the nineties. *Journal of Community Education* 8 (2) 12–16.

Percy, K. (1990a) Opinions, facts, and hypotheses: older adults and participation in learning activities in the United Kingdom. In Glendenning, F. and Percy, K. (eds) *Ageing, Education and Society. Readings in Educational Gerontology,* Keele: The University, Keele, Staffs, ST5 5BG.

Percy, K. (1990b) The future of education gerontology: a second statement of first principals. In: Glendenning, F. and Percy, K. (eds) *Ageing, Education and Society. Readings in Educational Gerontology,* Keele: The University, Keele, Staffs, ST5 5BG.

Scales, A.M. and Biggs, S.A. (1987) Reading habits of elderly adults: implications for instruction. *Educational Gerontology* 13, 521–532.

Thompson, J. (1987) Ageing of the population: contemporary trends and issues, *Population Trends* 50, Office of Population Censuses and Surveys, London: HMSO.

Wenger, G.C. (1989) Support networks in old age: constructing a typology in Jefferys, M. (ed) *Growing Old in the Twentieth Century.* London and New York: Routledge.

Withnall, A. (1989) Research notes: talking with older people. *Journal of Educational Gerontology* 4, 37–40.

CHAPTER 4

Health and Ageing Within Ethnic Minorities

Shah Ebrahim

Ethnicity and Health

This chapter is concerned with the demographic changes affecting elderly people in Britain from the 'visible' ethnic groups (Afro-Caribbean and Asians*), and the implications of these changes both for ageing individuals, and for health care systems. In addition to this focus upon health, accompanying social issues, together with their underlying determinants, will also be considered. Finally, having identified particular problems, some possible solutions for the future will be discussed.

Ethnicity

Ethnicity is not a clear cut categorical variable about which there can be no doubt. Ethnicity embraces religious, geographic, linguistic, cultural, and migratory differences between people, as well as place of birth (Fennell *et al* 1988). The simplistic approach of asking about country of birth is clearly a crude approximation of the truth. Amongst elderly people however it is probably a better approximation than amongst young adults, many of whom may have been born, and have parents who were also born, in the UK.

The term 'immigrant' is now rarely used, and the concepts of second and third generation immigrants are viewed as divisive, although the racial disadvantage that goes along with being visibly different from the majority is not a redundant concept. Research in this area has undergone semantic change as ideas and sensitivities have changed (Markides and Mindel 1987). This means that the definitions and criteria used for classification must be closely examined in reviews of previous work (Donovan 1984).

In Britain, the 1981 census dealt with the definition of ethnicity by simply asking about country of birth, without asking about parents' country of birth (as the previous, 1971, census had done). The size of the various ethnic populations is probably a substantial underestimate of true sizes because of under-completion of this question. Tests of an ethnic question were con-

---

* Here 'Asian' refers to those originating from the Indian subcontinent e.g. India, Pakistan, and Bangladesh.

ducted prior to the census and demonstrated enormous antipathy towards the concept of ethnicity or race, and problems of classification of people who held British passports and had the right of residence in the UK, but who had black or brown skin (OPCS 1978, 1980).

The 1991 census will classify people according to country of origin: Indian, Pakistani, Bangladeshi, 'other Asian', Black Caribbean, Black African. This too will present problems for people who consider themselves to be Black British. Substantial effort was put into ensuring high response rates amongst ethnic groups, particularly in inner cities, since the levels of government support depend ultimately on population sizes.

Although the populations shown in Figure 4.1 are small, it is clear that the 40–60/65 age group is much larger and will lead to large relative increases in the numbers of ethnic elders over the next 20–30 years. The rates of increase will be much larger than amongst the white population, although the absolute numbers of ethnic elders will be tiny compared with the white population. For example, in Nottingham (population of around 400,000) the number of Asian pensioners is around 300, and this will rise to about 900 over the next 20 years.

A further problem in much published research is the use of the term 'Asian'. South Asia is a big place, and there is a world of difference between

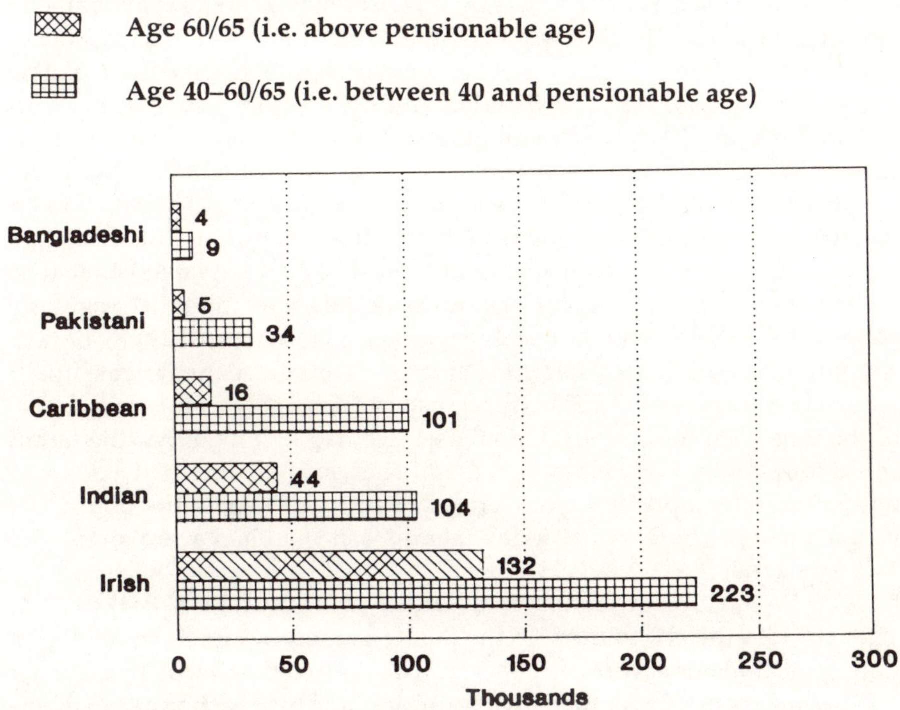

Source: OPCS, 1981

Figure 4.1: Numbers of Ethnic Elders in Great Britain (1981 Census)

Gujarat and Bangladesh. To group such populations together is a nonsense and is unlikely to lead to a better understanding of the influence of ethnicity on health and the process of ageing.

Myths

Any minority community that is not well understood generates myths both in its own and the host community. These myths serve functions for both communities – they demystify, they make life more tolerable, they allow subtle discrimination to continue. A prevalent host community myth, for example, concerns the supportive role of the extended family – 'they look after their own'. This is a powerful means of ignoring the needs of single people and couples. A survey in Birmingham demonstrated that, amongst the Afro-Caribbean elders, almost a third lived alone, and among the Asian elders, one in twenty lived alone, with a quarter living as couples (Blakemore 1982, 1983). The myth of extended family care is one reason why domiciliary services and community nursing services are so seldom provided for Asian elders.

A family doctor colleague tells a story about care in the community if you are Bangladeshi. A Bangladeshi woman had a stroke which left her badly paralysed and unable to speak. A social worker saw the family, and her children were used as interpreters, as no hospital interpreter was available. The family was asked if they would be able to take her home that week. They replied with a literal reply: 'Yes, they would be able to take their mother home'. What they meant was that they could physically transport her from hospital to home. They had a moral duty to take her home – that they were sure of. What they were not sure of, and what they were never asked, was whether they would manage to care for their mother properly. Much to the delight of the hospital staff she went home. It was a 'successful' discharge, but for the family it was a nightmare. No-one had explained that their mother would be incontinent and must be taken to the toilet regularly. No-one told them how to keep her mobile. No-one told them how to communicate with a dysphasic person. When the patient was finally referred for advice, she was bed-fast, had pressure sores, and wailed most of the time. The community nursing service had assumed that the family could cope – there were enough of them. The social services had a policy of not providing support if there were other people living in the house. The hospital had not bothered to follow her up – she had had a stroke, so what could be done?

A myth that afflicts ethnic elders is the myth of the return (Barker 1984). The return to the old country, to the family home – but a return in glory is important. Economic pressures were major forces for most migrants in persuading them to leave their own countries. To return with ample evidence of success is feasible, to return as poor as one left the country is not permissible. And yet the myth of the return is a powerful image of hope that one day sufficient money will be put aside to return. It is also a reason for not making provision for an old age in the host country.

A patient on a long-stay hospital ward had suffered a bad stroke and was effectively bed-fast. She was in her seventies and had a large family. They visited often, but over the years she lived in the hospital she became more and more withdrawn. She was barely awake most days but seemed in a daze. The family finally decided to buy the air tickets and took her to a nursing home in her own home town. The flight was a major ordeal as the cabin crew had no idea how badly disabled their passenger was. However, within a week of resettlement she was better than the family had seen her in years. The return was no myth and had worked a minor miracle.

Further myths are to do with service use: if black and ethnic minority groups do not use a service, then they do not need it. Related to this is the idea that if their problems were really bad they would use the present services, and that health and social services are open to all comers irrespective of race or culture (the 'colour-blind' approach). Ethnic elders, in common with the general elderly population, are too often viewed as a 'problem' that requires a 'solution', and it is easy to fall into the trap of considering their health service use as the problem, rather than their underlying ill-health.

Assimilation

Ethnic minority studies have largely concentrated on the responses of younger people to migration and assimilation (Khan 1979, Watson 1977, Rose 1969). However, more recent work has examined the relationships between ethnicity and ageing, exploring the extent to which assimilation occurs (Driedger and Chappell 1987). American studies have emphasised the importance of generational differences in the process of adjustment and assimilation to the host society (Guns 1979, Markides and Mindel 1987). The belief that assimilation of diverse ethnic groups into a host culture may be used as a justification to leave ethnic elders' special needs unmet. However, in Canada, where the two major ethnic groups – French and English speaking – have lived together for generations, the evidence points to continued differences. Separate nursing homes and day centres have been set up to cater for these different Canadian communities (Driedger and Chappell 1987).

Nevertheless, ethnic minority communities are in a transition. People who came to Britain to earn money to send home have entered a phase of consolidation, when kin join them, and families are built up. The 'sojouners' have become 'settlers'.

Ethnicity and Patterns of Disease

The history of medical interest in ethnicity has been described elsewhere (Johnson 1984). Early concerns were with 'exotic' imported diseases and

'Port Medicine'; there followed interest in genetic susceptibility as measured by 'race'; and more recently a literature on service provision has emerged.

Mortality

The most important information on patterns of disease comes from examination of mortality data, using routine details from death certificates for the numerator, and census data for the denominators in the calculation of rates (Marmot *et al* 1984). This approach relies on place of birth as a proxy for ethnicity, but is powerful because large numbers of events are considered.

Overall death rates at younger ages are almost invariably lower among any migrant group than either the host population, or the country the group comes from. This is explained by the healthy migrant effect; people have to be relatively healthy to migrate in the first place, and this is reflected in their lower death rates. As these populations age it is much less likely that the healthy migrant effect will continue to operate, and it is much more likely that the adverse social, economic and environmental factors experienced by migrants will take their toll, and be expressed as higher death rates.

A different picture emerges when death from particular causes is examined. In such analyses the common causes of death amongst Asians aged 20–74 are tuberculosis, diabetes, ischaemic heart disease, and motor vehicle accidents, but cancer deaths are rare. Caribbean people have a similar pattern of mortality with the exception that death rates for hypertensive disease are remarkably high, and usually associated with stroke. In contrast, ischaemic heart disease and motor vehicle accidents are less common than expected (Adelstein and Marmot 1989).

Morbidity

Death rates only give part of the story, and tell us nothing about chronic diseases that only rarely cause death. Routine data on morbidity are rare, but the hospital activity analysis system does give place of birth together with diagnosis at discharge from hospital. This information has been used to compare the discharge rate ratios of elderly people born in the UK and in South Asia and the Caribbean (Ebrahim *et al* 1987). High rates for diabetes, asthma, and gastro-intestinal bleeding were observed for Asians, together with very high rates for cataract surgery. High notification rates for tuberculosis are found in all ethnic groups (Medical Research Council 1980).

In the population at large, a single study of Asian elders in Leicester has been reported (Donaldson 1986). This survey demonstrated high levels of disability in activities of daily living (ability to bathe, use the toilet, etc.), but no group of white elders of similar age and social background was available for comparison. Furthermore, it is difficult to know whether the high levels of disability were determined by physical or mental illness or social factors, such as perceived danger of walking outdoors, method of bathing, the adverse environment of the inner city, etc. Disability may differ in its cultural perception, particularly among people who have had limited experience of long-term degenerative diseases. Little work has been done in this area.

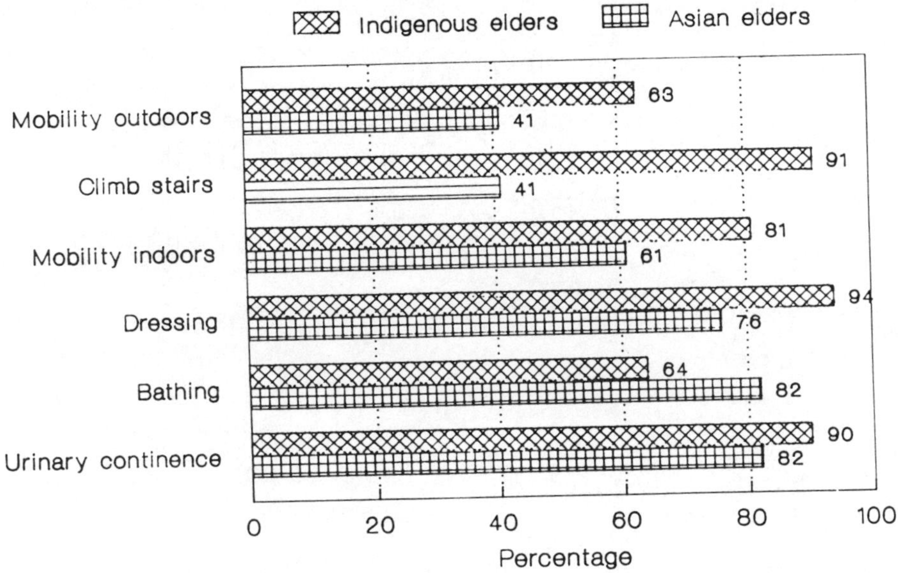

Source: Donaldson, BMJ, 1986

Figure 4.2: Ethnicity and disability among elderly people (75+) living in Leicester and Melton Mowbray, England

In primary health care, the high levels of consultation, particularly by Asians, have drawn comment, and there is a tendency to define this as a problem of 'over-utilization'. A comparative study of Gujarati Asians and age and sex matched white elders was recently reported by Ebrahim *et al* (1991). This study arose out of a local primary health care team's concern that despite high levels of consultation, Asian patients continued to attend, and yet seemed to derive little benefit. The study found that Asian elders had much higher levels of diagnosed disease and prescription drugs – thus explaining their high consultation rates – but were surprisingly less handicapped by their diseases. Life satisfaction levels were higher than in the white population!

Surveys of illness in Asian populations have typically ignored the elderly, probably because of their small numbers. However, consistent findings at younger ages are the excess of ischaemic heart disease in Asians, but not Afro-Caribbeans, and the increased risk of diabetes in both groups (Hughes *et al* 1989, Fox *et al* 1988, McKeigue *et al* 1989). Surprisingly, Afro-Caribbeans are at much greater risk of stroke than Asians.

Psychiatric illness rates are subject to much controversy, and particular attention has been drawn to the inappropriate application of usual criteria for diagnosis of psychotic illness across different cultures. Among Asians,

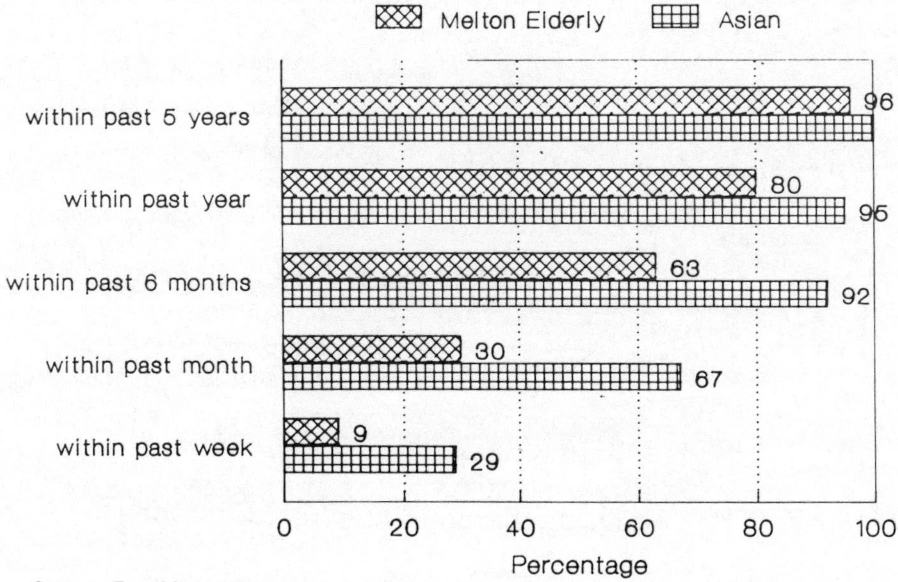

Source: Donaldson, 1986

Figure 4.3: GP consultations among indigenous (Melton) and Asian Elders living in Leicester, England

depression, anxiety states, and psychotic illness appear to be either as common, or less common than among the white population (Cochrane and Stopes-Roe 1981). Among Afro-Caribbeans it is possible that admission rates for schizophrenia are more common than expected (Cochrane 1977, 1979). However, the whole business of measuring illness rates in inner city populations is made extremely difficult because of shifting and inaccurate denominators (Burke 1989).

The explanation for these patterns of disease is likely to be a complex mix of environmental factors (including health behaviours, but also more general effects of poor housing and poverty), and genetic susceptibility. Marmot *et al* (1984) provide a useful classification for thinking about the reasons for differing patterns of disease in migrant populations: influences of the old country; influences of the new country; selection of who migrates; and the process of adaptation. For example, tuberculosis is a clear example of a disease that is common in South Asia and most warm climate countries; it is therefore more common amongst people from these countries. By contrast, ischaemic heart disease, diabetes and strokes are rare in rural areas of warm climate countries, but become very common amongst migrant populations. It appears that it is the transition from rural to urban location that is associated with the increased risk as these diseases are now relatively common among all social strata in the capital cities of South Asia. Selection effects at younger ages lead to the 'healthy migrant' effect, with migrants experiencing much lower overall death and disease rates than the population they come from. This is simply explained by the fact that people have to be fit to migrate in the first place, and such effects tend to wear off as the years pass. The process of adaptation has been used to explain differences in psychiatric illness.

Constructs of Health and Illness

The transition from high levels of infectious diseases, many of which are self-limiting regardless of medical care, to chronic degenerative disease, much of which may require long-term medication (e.g. diabetes, asthma, ischaemic heart disease) is likely to be associated with changes in ideas about the causation of illness, and what should be done to reduce its adverse effects.

Much of what is known about constructs of illness is derived from social anthropological research usually conducted in developing countries (see for example, Blanchet 1984, Gardner 1990), although increasingly work is being done in the UK (Eade 1990, McDonald 1987). The main illness models that have general currency are: the western medical model with its separation of physical and mental domains, and its emphasis on professional and technological intervention; religious models (Islamic, for example) emphasising a unification of body and mind, and understanding of disease (and cure) through divine intervention; folk/traditional models which usually emphasise the role of external forces (spirits, sorcery) in disease causation; and a wide range of therapies (ranging from spirit ceremonies to herbal treatments).

The non-western medical models offer a non-victim blaming approach for the causation of disease, whereas western views are increasingly concerned with health behaviours (smoking, diet, exercise) that influence risk of disease and may be controlled by the individual. Religious and traditional views tend to emphasise the importance of living in balance with other unpredictable surrounding forces, and the avoidance of potentially dangerous situations which may lead to exposure to spirits or sorcery. These differences in perspective are by no means fixed, and it is typical for people to move easily from one model of illness and healing to another. An awareness of such behaviour is relevant in discussing illness with ethnic elders, since most people have a general unwillingness to talk about traditional beliefs, perhaps for fear of being thought superstitious or stupid.

Use of Health and Social Services

In old age, under-reporting of symptoms and under-identification of disease by practitioners both occur. Often, problems such as incontinence, foot problems, depression, hearing and visual impairments are not known of by family doctors. It is likely that this is because of the poor availability of treatment, the belief that action will not be helpful, and that the overall benefits will not outweigh the costs. In addition, individuals vary widely in their perception of symptoms such as pain, and in their notion of what is a significant disease. It is probable that these factors all play a part in the use made by ethnic elders of existing services.

Health Care and Community Services

Ethnic elders are high users of general practitioner and hospital services but have low use of community nursing and social services, particularly meals on wheels and home helps (Barker 1984, Blakemore 1982, 1983, Balarajan *et al* 1989, Gillam *et al* 1989). Despite high levels of health service use, it would be wrong to conclude that all is well. It is quite possible that access to the service is not a problem, but that the quality of care and outcomes of care are substantially worse. No systematic information is available to support or refute these hypotheses. In a small study, while hospital admission was much more common among Asian elders, follow-up in an outpatient clinic was much less frequent (Ebrahim *et al* 1991). This implies that hospital teams are less likely to offer follow-up for Asian patients (perhaps because of an unwillingness to see people who don't speak English in a clinic that does not have an interpreter), which may indicate a lower quality of care.

Hospitals tend to focus on obvious areas such as interpreters, meals, numbers of visitors allowed, signs and patient information in appropriate languages (Henley 1979). While such aspects of the hospital are important for ethnic elders, they are not substitutes for the employment of people from local ethnic communities, nor for adequate advocacy for elderly people.

In practice, the amount of advocacy work that goes on for any ethnic group is extremely limited. Chronically disabled ethnic elders frequently do not appear to get the support and help that their disabilities would suggest is needed. As already described, it is commonplace for people to be discharged rapidly after a stroke with the assumption that the family will cope. Yet all too frequently the family is not told about the management of, say, a urinary catheter, or how to feed someone who is prone to choke, or the opportunities (limited though they are) for respite care.

Managers of community home care services that are not used by ethnic elders may feel that this is appropriate because of extensive family support. While generally unhelpful, this major myth does have some basis in fact; a majority of ethnic elders do live in extended family groups – but not all. Presumably those on their own are likely to need home care support, but may find the standard style of service unacceptable, inappropriate, or may simply not know they are eligible.

Day centres and lunch clubs for mixed ethnicity groups are rare; in general elders prefer to mix with people from their own backgrounds. This applies both between major ethnic divisions and also within groups. For example, while Caribbean people may look similar, the identity and culture of places like Jamaica and St Lucia are very different. Elders from these places may resent the idea that they have anything in common and may be unwilling to use the same club. However, other individuals may find the cultural diversity and atmosphere in an Afro-Caribbean elders club stimulating. It is clearly wrong to make any assumptions about what ethnic elders may or may not find acceptable.

The most widely desired community service in most inner city areas is a day centre, and many ethnic groups have great difficulty in achieving this. Day centres are an important community resource, and permit a wide range of other activities that benefit the housebound and carers. High priority must be given to providing facilities and training to run day centres for ethnic elders. Most of these centres are presently run by the voluntary sector (with minimal support) indicating how little priority statutory local authority services have placed on developing this aspect of provision. It is easy to see why local councils do not build (or convert) day centres for ethnic elders: it is very unpopular with white voters (and poll tax payers) and several schemes in London have fallen under local opposition.

Jeopardy

The triple jeopardy hypothesis of ethnic minority ageing is a useful starting point for examining what happens to ethnic elders (Norman 1985). Elders are at jeopardy because of their ethnicity – racial discrimination. The second jeopardy is by virtue of their age, and the third is due to socio-economic disadvantage. For elderly Asian women it seems obvious to add a fourth jeopardy to this list: female sex. The purdah of Islam is perhaps the most apparent example of the limited life of many Asian women. The impact of these several jeopardies could lead to worse health and more limited use of health and social services.

A double jeopardy hypothesis was put forward earlier, and predicts an adverse interaction between getting older (the first jeopardy) and belonging to an ethnic minority (the second jeopardy [Moore 1971]). The alternative hypothesis, that a lifetime of prejudice and discrimination is an excellent grounding for old age, has been stated (Dowd and Bengtson 1978), and is linked to the notion of the levelling effects of old age. The double jeopardy hypothesis can be extended by adding other jeopardies, made easy by the multi-dimensional nature of ageing and ethnicity.

The evidence presented in this review demonstrates that ethnic elders are certainly very vulnerable to the impact of age-related diseases, that the social support they receive is markedly less than they appear to require, and that, although access to health care is not a problem, subsequent processes and outcomes of care are not known.

What Changes are Needed?

Primary care

Primary care is central to improving the health of ethnic elders. At present, great use is made of the general practitioner, and a greater emphasis on ensuring that these contacts are productive is needed. This may mean employing staff from the local ethnic community to ensure that communication is feasible. A prevention programme is clearly needed to reduce the burden of disease associated with common diseases. Collaboration with health authority health promotion staff will usually locate relevant material and ideas.

The general practitioner is also in a good position to become a patient's advocate, asking questions about quality of care, and ensuring that requests for re-housing and for welfare benefits advice are channelled to the right places.

Community care

With extensive changes in the organisation of community care currently underway in Britain, it is possible that the Local Authorities (the present managers of state social care) will cease to be the major providers of services for elderly people, and particularly for ethnic elders. The idea of 'contracting out' the provision of Halal meals on wheels, for example, could prove very popular with Local Authorities who have failed to organise their own service in the past.

However, a major barrier to achieving more appropriate services organised by an independent (either profit making or voluntary) sector is that such facilities are not common in inner city areas. Over the last 20 years various groups have argued a strong case for main stream funding for services for ethnic communities. The present independent sector policy may not be accepted as the right solution by many local communities.

Even if there is agreement that the local ethnic communities should take a part in providing services (e.g. good neighbour schemes, night sitting services, home care services, meals, day centres), a considerable amount of training will be required. Greater levels of trust between local authorities and the existing voluntary agencies will be needed, and a commitment to provide secure funding and premises will be essential.

References

Adelstein, A.M. and Marmot, M.G. (1989) The health of migrants in England and Wales: causes of death. In Cruickshank, J.K. and Beevers, D.G., (eds) *Ethnic Factors in Health and Disease.* London: Wright.

Balarajan, R., Yuen, P. and Raleigh, V.S. (1989) Ethnic differences in general practitioner consultations. *British Medical Journal* 299, 958–60.

Barker, J. (1984) *Black and Asian old people in Britain.* Mitcham: Age Concern Research Unit.

Blakemore, K. (1982) Health and illness among the elderly of minority ethnic groups living in Birmingham: some new findings. *Health Trends* 14, 69–72.

Blakemore, K. (1983) Ethnicity, self-reported illness and use of medical services by the elderly. Postgraduate Medical Journal 59, 668–70.

Blanchet, T. (1984) *Meanings and rituals of birth in rural Bangladesh.* Dhaka: University Press.

Bulmer, M. (1988) Race and Ethnicity. In Burgess R.C. (ed) *Key Variables in Social Investigation.* London: Routledge and Kegan Paul.

Burke, A. (1989) Psychiatric practice and ethnic minorities. In Cruickshank, J.K. and Beevers, D.G., (eds) *Ethnic Factors in Health and Disease.* London: Wright.

Cochrane, R. (1977) Mental illness in immigrants to England and Wales. *Social Psychiatry* 12, 25–37.

Cochrane, R. (1979) Psychological and behavioural disturbance in West Indians, Indians and Pakistanis in Britain: a comparison of rates among children and adults. *British Journal of Psychiatry* 134, 201–10.

Cochrane, R. and Stopes-Roe, M. (1981) Psychological symptom levels in Indian immigrants to England – a comparison with native English. *Psychological Medicine,* 11, 319–27.

Donaldson, L. (1986) Health and social status of elderly Asians: a community survey. *British Medical Journal* 293, 1079–82.

Donovan, J. (1984) Ethnicity and health – a research review. *Social Science and Medicine* 19, 663–70.

Dowd, J.J. and Bengtson, V.L. (1978) Ageing in minority populations: an examination of the double jeopardy hypothesis. *Journal of Gerontology* 33, 427–36.

Driedger, L. and Chappell, N. (1987) *Aging and Ethnicity: Towards an Interface.* Toronto: Butterworths.

Eade, J. (1990) Bangladeshi community organisation and leadership in Tower Hamlets East London. In Clarke, C., Peach, C. and Vertovec, S. (eds) *South Asians Overseas: Migration and Ethnicity,* Cambridge: Cambridge University Press.

Ebrahim, S., Smith, C. and Giggs, J. (1987) Elderly immigrants – a disadvantaged group? *Age and Ageing* 16, 249–55.

Ebrahim, S., Patel, N., Coats, M. *et al* (1991) Prevalence and severity of morbidity among Gujarati Asian elders: a controlled comparison. *Family Practice* 8, 57–62.

Fennell, G., Phillipson, C., Evers H. (1988) Race, Ethnicity and Old Age. In *The Sociology of Old Age.* Milton Keynes: Open University Press.

Fox, K.M. and Shapiro, L.M. (1988) Heart disease in Asians in Britain. *British Medical Journal* 297, 311–2.

Gardner, K. (1990) Keeping the world in order: exorcism and healing in rural Bangladesh. Unpublished PhD thesis. London School of Economics.

Gillam, S.J., Jarman, B., White, P. and Law, R. (1989) Ethnic differences in consultation rates in urban general practice. *British Medical Journal* 299, 953–7.

Guns, H. (1979) Symbolic ethnicity: the future of ethnic groups and cultures in America. *Ethnic and Racial Studies* 2, 1–20.

Henley, A. (1979) *Asian patients in hospital and at home.* London: Kings Fund.

Hughes, L.O., Cruickshank, J.K., Wright, J. and Raferty, E.B. (1989) Disturbances of insulin in British Asian and white men surviving myocardial infarction. *British Medical Journal* 299, 537–41.

Johnson, M.R.C. (1984) Ethnic Minorities and Health. *Journal of the Royal College of Physicians of London* 18, 228–230.

Khan, V.S. (1979) Migration and Social Stress: Murpuris in Bradford. In Khan V.S. (ed) *Minority Families in Britain.* London: MacMillan.

Markides, K.S. and Mindel, C.H. (1987) *Aging and Ethnicity.* Newbury Park: Sage.

McDonald, M. (1987) Rituals of motherhood among Gujarati women in East London. In: Burghart (ed) *Hinduism in Great Britain: The Perpetuation of Religion in an Alien Cultural Milieu,* London: Tavistock.

McKeigue, P.M., Miller, G.J. and Marmot, M.G. (1989) Coronary heart disease in South Asians overseas – a review. *Journal of Clinical Epidemiology* 42, 597–609.

Marmot, M., Adelstein, A.M. and Bulusi, L. (1984) Immigrant mortality in England and Wales (1970–78): causes of death by country. *OPCS Studies of Medical and Population Subjects* (47). London: HMSO.

Medical Research Council, Tuberculosis and Chest Disease Unit (1980) National Survey of Tuberculosis notifications in England and Wales, 1978–79. *British Medical Journal* 286, 895–8.

Moore, J.W. Situational factors affecting minority ageing. *Gerontologist* 11, 88–92.

Norman, A. (1985) *Triple jeopardy: growing old in a second homeland.* London: Centre for Policy on Ageing.

Office of Population Censuses and Surveys Monitor 1981 Census (1978) *Developing a question on ethnic origin (CEN 78/4).* London: HMSO.

Office of Population Censuses and Surveys Monitor 1981 Census (1980) *Tests of an ethnic question (CEN 80/3).* London: HMSO.

Office of Population Censuses and Surveys (1983) *Census 1981, Country of Birth; Great Britain.* London: HMSO.

Rose, E.J.B. (1969) *Colour and Citizenship.* Oxford: OUP / Institute of Race Relations.

Watson, J.L. (1977) *Between two cultures: migrants and minorities in Britain,* Oxford: Blackwell.

CHAPTER 5

The Transmission of Income Inequality
Gender and Non-state Pensions

Jay Ginn and Sara Arber

Demographic change has spurred debate about ageing and the elderly in recent years, a debate dominated by over-generalised stereotypes of elderly people. They are variously portrayed as poor and disadvantaged (the social problem view), as fit, active and independent (the optimistic view), or as a burden on the rest of society. These views are ageist, in that a set of characteristics is attributed solely on the basis of age. They fail to reflect the wide differences among elderly people in income, health and lifestyle.

This chapter shows how such ageist conceptions, by assuming homogeneity, obscure class and gender inequalities, and the part played by political and social processes in creating them. Inequalities in personal income among elderly people are examined, focussing on the sources of gender inequality of income. We assess the impact of the sexual division in the labour market and of women's roles in the domestic economy on pension income in later life.

Ageism – Three Variants

1. Compassionate Ageism

The contrasting ageist views about elderly people may be summarised as follows. The first, the longstanding and familiar 'social problem' view, focusses on the multiple disadvantages of old age, ranging from the material constraints of poverty and disability to social devaluation, role loss and isolation. Commentators have dwelt on the problems of elderly people, on the inadequacy of state benefits and of medical and social services to meet their needs, and on the plight of informal carers. This problem-centred approach has been termed 'compassionate ageism', reflecting its good intentions to ameliorate poverty and ill-health, but also its stereotyping of elderly people (Minkler 1984, 16).

An emphasis on the problems experienced by elderly people is a legitimate concern, especially for those closely involved in the development of services and provision of care. But where writers focus on the disadvantages of old age, they can contribute to a stereotype of elderly people as weak, dependent and burdensome. The danger arises of presenting a partial, one-dimensional view, which defines elderly people as a social problem, reinforces the low esteem in which they are held, condescends to them as objects of welfare, and ignores diversity.

2. *The Optimistic Alternative*

A more recent 'optimistic' view of elderly people highlights the expansion of opportunities for leisure, consumption, personal development, and contribution to society during retirement, and reminds us of the independence and good health of the majority of elderly people (Laslett 1987; Wells and Freer 1988). In its most extreme form (Fries 1980), the optimistic view predicts the 'rectangularisation of mortality'. Instead of the survival rate decreasing gradually from age 65, it would remain stable at a high level until 85 (the age claimed to represent the limit of the natural life span), when it would fall steeply. Thus an increasing proportion of the population would live to 85 years of age, but few would survive beyond this. An important corollary is the prediction of a 'compression of morbidity'; an increasing proportion of elderly people would remain free of disease or disability until a short illness precipitates death. In this scenario increased longevity means a prolongation of active, worthwhile life. Far from being a problem, it is cause for celebration.

Although individual variation is recognised, the optimistic view tends to overlook the differences in health and life expectancy by class and gender, and the improbability of these disappearing without radical political and social change.

3. *Conflictual Ageism*

A third variant, which we have termed 'conflictual ageism', depicts pensioners as a financially secure and politically powerful group, who are imposing an unjustifiable and increasingly costly burden on the rest of society through their consumption of pensions and health and welfare services (Binstock 1984; Minkler 1986). While this view is not new, it has seen a resurgence in the 1980s, and has contributed to a 'moral panic' about the ageing of populations in industrial societies. Its proponents, who are more political than sociological, and include Americans for Generational Equity (AGE), prophesy an 'age war' between generations, and blame poverty among families with children on excessive consumption of resources by elderly people (Longman 1987). As one British journalist put it, '...the over 60's are our nouveaux rich' (Paterson 1988).

A recent British book to sound an alarm over the expansion in numbers and increasing burden on society of elderly people is *Workers Versus Pensioners: Intergenerational Justice in an Ageing World* (Johnson *et al* 1989), a collection of contributions whose theme is the impending conflict over resources between pensioners and succeeding cohorts throughout the industrial world. Like the 'conflictual ageism' expressed by AGE, this thesis maintains that while pensioners enjoy unprecedented affluence, welfare benefits for those in earlier stages of the life cycle are being cut. This, together with the changing demographic balance between workers and pensioners will, it is argued, bring about intergenerational conflict over taxation and benefits, unless circumvented by policies encouraging later retirement or by a reduction in the value of pensions.

Gerontologists and sociologists have taken issue with several aspects of this argument (for example, see Phillipson 1990, Greene 1989). But it is the neglect of income inequality among elderly people in all three ageist views that we wish to challenge here, and especially the way that class and gender divisions are overlooked.

Pensioners' Income – Poverty or Affluence?

The claim of increasing relative affluence among pensioners is a strange one where British pensioners are concerned; the slight relative improvement in mean income between 1960 and 1982 was mainly due to the rise of unemployment and cuts in social security payment levels to other groups (Walker 1986, Phillipson 1990) and left a substantial income gap between elderly people and the population as a whole. The mean disposable income of those aged 65 to 74, adjusted for family size, is 76% of the mean for all ages, while that of people 75 or over is only 67% (Hedstrom and Ringen 1987).

More fundamentally, quoting mean income serves to mask inequalities among pensioners arising from their previous labour market and domestic experiences, and ignores the increasing inequality of their incomes (Bradshaw and O'Higgins 1984). Ageist generalisations about pensioners which ignore gender or previous occupation are misleading in view of the evidence emerging from research which demonstrates that the social divisions of working life are carried over into old age.

Arber (1989) has shown that for male pensioners previous occupation is a major determinant of the source and amount of their income. Middle class people in retirement are both wealthier and healthier than their working class counterparts. They are more likely to have occupational pensions, and to own their homes (Evandrou and Victor 1989). The ways in which gender, as well as class, contributes to the structuring of inequality of income in later life is discussed at greater length below.

Retirement – Imposed or Chosen?

The tendency to discuss elderly people as if they were a homogeneous group is also evident in the debate over the nature and causes of dependency in old age. On the one hand it is argued that elderly people are the victims of 'structured dependency', having been forced into a dependent and marginalised position by social policies which exclude them from the labour market (Townsend 1981). On the other hand Johnson (1989) maintains that the fall in age of retirement during this century reflects employees' choice to leave work, and that dependency on the vagaries of the labour market is just as real and oppressive as that on state benefits.

But the experience of retirement is socially divided. Retirement, like work, may be experienced as either a blessing or a curse, depending mainly on two factors which both vary according to class and gender. First, the income available from pensions and other sources, the assets acquired, and the standard of living which can be maintained; and second, the nature of the work situation, whether providing opportunities for rewarding activities and social contact, or whether an alienating, stressful burden, taking its toll on health and vitality.

The constraint imposed by low pension income is no less now than a generation ago:

> Freedom of choice between work and retirement is not meaningful if prospective retirement income is seriously inadequate (Gordon 1963 p.457).

Walker points out the class-divided nature of retirement:

> There are those, mainly salaried workers, who are able to choose whether or not to leave work at the retirement age... Then there are those, predominantly manual workers, who are effectively coerced into retirement and sometimes early retirement by poor working conditions, ill-health, redundancy and unemployment (Walker 1986 p.10).

Class differences in the likelihood and cause of 'premature exit' from the labour market for men are shown by Arber (1989) using data from the 1980–1982 General Household Survey (GHS). Among those who have left the labour force before 65, early retirement (implying choice) is more common among professionals, managers and employers, whereas exit because of disability or unemployment (implying lack of choice) is primarily among manual workers. Thus the privilege of choosing when to retire may be as unequally distributed by class as are wealth and income.

Gender as well as class affects the circumstances of retirement. For older women, additional constraints on the choice of continuing in employment arise from the expectation that they will fulfil caring roles for a husband or older relatives and that they will retire at the same time as their husbands (Joshi 1987 p.112). An intensive study of 18 long-married couples aged between 50 and 70 found that:

> It was taken for granted by the couples that the wives would either retire before their husbands or at the same time; they would or should

not continue in paid employment longer than their husbands (Mason 1987 p.96).

Gender Differences in Life Contributions and Rewards

The gender dimension of poverty has been generally neglected in research (Glendinning and Millar 1987). This omission is especially glaring in later life, when the population is predominantly female. Peace (1986 p.61) refers to 'the forgotten female', noting that 'old women are all around us and yet invisible', their existence and their needs rarely acknowledged in spite of their numbers.

Where the concentration of poverty among elderly women has been recognized, it has been explained in terms of the failings of the social security system, while 'The social and economic factors which had caused these women to have inadequate resources in the first place were simply not considered' (Millar and Glendinning 1989 p.368). Studies of income in later life generally fail to examine gender differences in detail or to consider how they may be related to pre-retirement experience, and to gender-bias in social policy, employment practice, and allocation of domestic responsibilities. Notable exceptions include Walker (1987), and Groves (1987). The latter argues that gender disadvantage is perpetuated into later life by the way state and occupational pension schemes operate. Arber shows that there is continuity from position in the occupational class structure during adult life into standard of living in later life, but also warns:

> Gender inequalities in the likelihood of receiving occupational pensions, the size of those pensions, and the ability to accumulate capital during the working life, may result in *increasing* gender inequality among the elderly in the future. This is particularly likely if the provision of personal occupational pensions is promoted and replaces the state retirement pension as the main means of financial support for the elderly (Arber 1989 p.95, our emphasis)

We argue that to understand the concentration of poverty among elderly women the idea of continuity must be extended to include the individual's position in the unpaid ('reproductive') economy as well as in the paid ('productive') economy during earlier stages of the life course. The unpaid domestic responsibilities of 'houseworkers' (Martin and Roberts 1984), mainly married women, reproduce society on a daily basis, by servicing and supporting male partners, and on a generational basis, by bearing and rearing children. These contributions by women to the continuation of society and to the welfare of kin are disadvantageous to women themselves, contributing to the cycle of their educational, training and occupational disadvantage which has been fully discussed by feminists and other writers (Caplow 1954, Klein 1965, Oakley 1974). There are two analytically distinct ways in which continuity of disadvantage for women may occur. The first is associated with marital status and motherhood, and the second with gender inequalities in the labour market.

1. Discontinuous and Part-time Employment

Earning a good occupational pension is facilitated by working continuously with one employer, since most schemes are non-transferable, and by maintaining full-time employment, since many employers restrict access to their scheme through an age limit, a length of service requirement, or a minimum hours threshold (Labour Research Department 1988). Continuous full-time employment is difficult to achieve for women with caring responsibilities towards children, husbands and other relatives (Martin and Roberts 1984; Petrie and Logan 1986; Joshi 1987) under existing conditions in Britain. Women are under pressure to leave work or switch to lower paid part-time work when they have children because of the unequal division of domestic labour and the notorious lack of government policies to provide or promote adequate child-care facilities. As a result, over a quarter of British women of working age in 1988 were employed part-time, a higher proportion than in any other European country.

Where part-time employees are allowed to join occupational pension schemes, their low wages ensure a substantially reduced occupational pension. Even where full-time work is eventually resumed after a career break, discontinuity both delays career progression, so that the final salary is on average lower than that of continuously employed women (Joshi 1987), and reduces the number of contribution years.

The amount of state pension which women can earn is also affected by their position in the domestic economy in several ways. First, where part-time wages are below the lower earnings limit (£46.00 per week in 1990), contributions are not payable, and 'qualifying years' are lost. Second, the low level of part-time wages limits the amount of state Graduated Pension and State Earnings Related Pension (SERPS), which can be earned. Third, career breaks reduce the number of years in which National Insurance (NI) basic (and additional earnings-related) contributions can be made. The introduction of Home Responsibilities Protection (HRP) credits in 1978 implied government recognition of the problem of career breaks due to caring responsibiliies. Those who cannot work because they are caring for a dependant are allowed a reduction in the required number of years to qualify for the N.I. pension. However, HRP does not compensate for the lower wages of part-time employees and the consequent reduction of SERPS entitlement. Fourth, the assumption by policy-makers of married women's dependency was manifested, from 1948 until 1978, in the married woman's right to exemption from the pension-earning part of N.I. contributions. Many married women chose exemption, forfeiting the right to their own NI pension.

For all these reasons 'for the foreseeable future... a considerable number [of women] will retire without a pension in their own right' (Dex and Phillipson 1986 p.56). Thus the capacity of women to obtain an adequate occupational or state earnings-related pension, or even a basic state pension in their own right, is constrained by the unpaid domestic provisioning and caring work they undertake for the benefit of others. Graham's observation that 'for women, economic dependency is the cost of caring' applies not only during working life, but also in retirement (Graham 1987 p.223).

2. *Gender Divisions in the Labour Market*

It is not only women with caring responsibilities who lose earnings and pension rights. The sexual division in the labour market, which is connected with social expectations about women's caring role, affects women of all ages and marital statuses. Women are concentrated within a narrow range of relatively low paid occupations and they also disproportionately occupy lower levels within organisations (Hakim 1979; Martin and Roberts 1984; Dex 1985). This occupational segregation, together with the undervaluing of 'women's work', has maintained women's average full-time pay at about two-thirds that of men, in spite of Equal Pay legislation.

Since the pension payable through schemes of all types (state basic, state earnings-related, occupational Final Salary, occupational Money Purchase, and privately arranged Personal Pension) depends on lifetime earnings, women have generally been unable to obtain as high an occupational or private pension as men, or to benefit fully from earnings-related state pension supplements. The loss of earnings and pension rights to which all women are exposed has been dubbed 'the price of being female' (Joshi 1987 p.130).

Thus, in spite of the increase in formal equality of the sexes, and of the steep increase during the last two decades in the economic activity rate among working-age women to 70%, retirement is not gender-neutral. The rules governing eligibility and levels of pensions have been geared to men's (middle class) patterns of employment and earnings. In combination with state policies which assume a breadwinning male and dependent female, pension arrangements discriminate against women.

Recent government policies have aimed to promote greater reliance on non-state pensions (occupational and private) as the main means of financial support of elderly people, a trend which is likely to increase income inequality in later life. In order to assess the magnitude of the effect of non-state pensions on gender inequality of income in the late 1980s, recent nationally representative data are analysed. A major aim is to measure the relative importance of attachment to domestic roles compared with gender *per se* – to quantify the 'cost of caring' as distinct from 'the price of being female'.

An Analysis of Data from the 1985 and 1986 General Household Survey

Combined data from the 1985 and 1986 General Household Survey (OPCS 1988, 1989) are analysed. With a response rate of 82% this provides high quality information about a nationally representative sample of over 7000 people over 65 years of age, living in private households in Britain.

The measure of income used here is the personal income to which an individual is entitled: we have not assumed equal sharing between spouses for two reasons. First, studies on distribution of resources within households (Pahl 1980, 1989, Edwards 1981, Evans 1983, Vogler 1989) have indicated that equal sharing cannot be assumed. Although it is likely that some redistribution occurs, especially between spouses, it is impossible to estimate the amounts of income flows. Second, when one spouse is financially dependent on the other, and her access to money is discretionary, it is perceived and used differently from independent income (Sen 1984, Glendinning and Millar 1987, Popay 1989). For example, Mason (1987) found that where wives in her sample of long-married couples had not 'earned' any pension income in their own right, all pension income was treated as belonging to the husband.

In the absence of information in the GHS on the childbearing history of elderly women, marital status is used as an indicator of degree of lifetime involvement in the domestic economy. Cohabiting couples are treated as married. The measure of class used in this analysis depends on the individual's last main occupation, using seven categories based on the Registrar General's socio-economic groups, with an additional category for those who have never been employed (see Appendix).

Gender Inequality in Income

The homogeneity implied by ageist conceptions of elderly people is not supported by national data on the distribution of personal income. The distribution of incomes for elderly women and men is shown in Figure 5.1 and two features of the distribution are noteworthy. First, within each gender there is a wide range of incomes (which, as we show later, is class-related). For instance, among men, 50% have a weekly income under £55.00, but 10% have more than twice as much (£121.00), and 1% have over £200.00. Second, gender makes a substantial difference to personal income, women's income distribution being not only lower than men's but flatter. Comparing women and men, the difference in weekly personal income is £16 at the median, £34 at the upper quartile, and £57 at the top decile.

Sources of Income for Elderly Women and Men

To understand gender inequality in income it is necessary to analyse whether it arises from a particular source of income. The income of elderly people

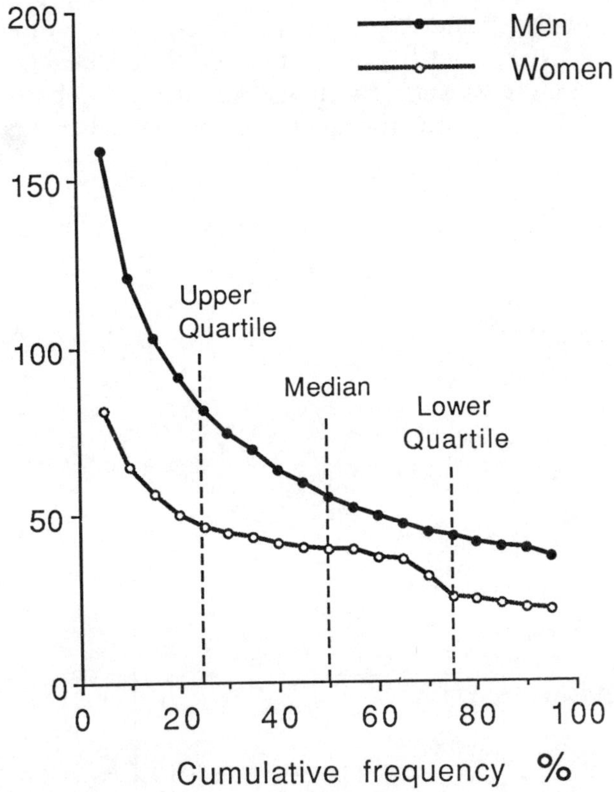

Source: General Household Survey 1985/86 (own analysis)

Figure 5.1: Distribution of total personal income in £s per week by gender

Table 5.1. Sources of income of elderly* men and women

Source	*% receiving income from each source*		
	Men	*Women*	*All*
State N.I.Pension	94	96	95
Supplementary Pension	7	15	12
Earnings	8	3	5
Interest on Savings	96	98	98
Payments from Friends/Relatives	<0.5	1	1
Other Regular Payments	1	<0.5	1
Occupational Pension (a)	62	26	40
Private Pension (b)	4	2	3
Non-state Pension (a and/or b)	64	27	42
Total	*2929*	*4340*	*7269*

* Elderly = people aged 65+
Source: General Household Survey 1985 and 1986 (own analysis)

comes from a variety of sources: the state, earnings, non-state pensions, and other sources of income such as interest, payments from friends and relatives. State benefits include National Insurance Retirement Pension, Supplementary Pension, and a range of need-related benefits (Invalidity Allowance, Widows Pension, Disability Allowance, Mobility Allowance, Attendance Allowance, and other short and long term benefits).

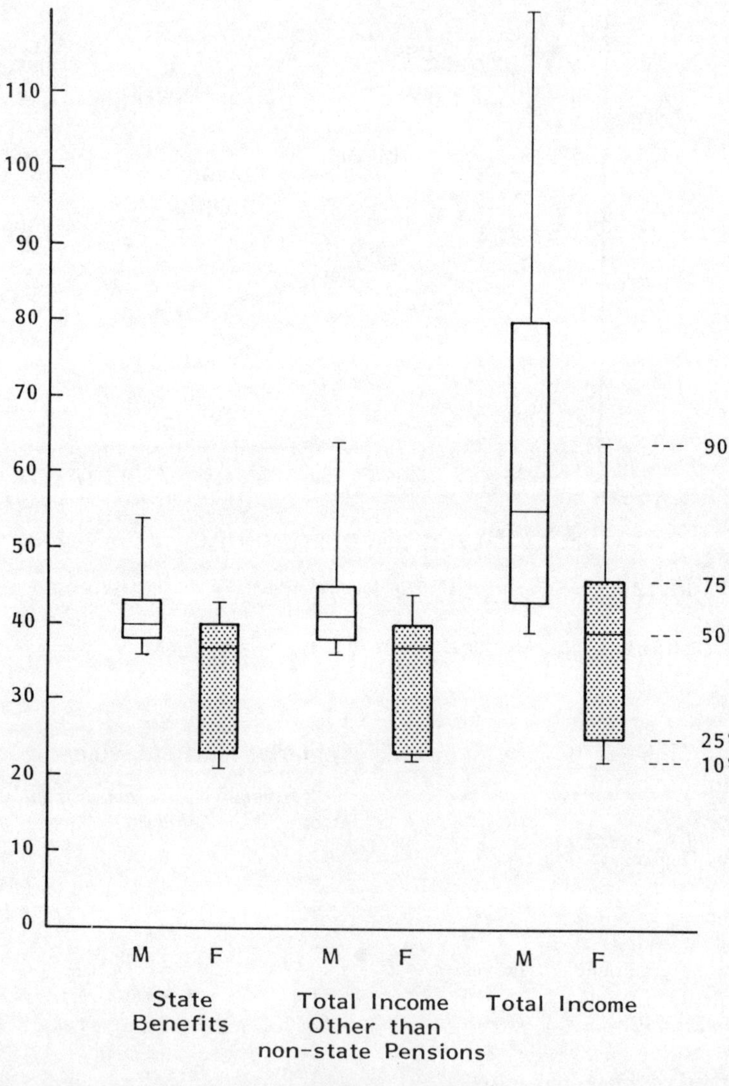

Source: General Household Survey 1985/86 (own analysis)

Figure 5.2: Distribution of income from different sources in £s per week by gender, N = 7269

Table 5.1 shows the percentage of elderly women and men receiving income from different sources. A much higher percentage of men than women have non-state pension income, 64% compared with 27%, and over twice as many men have earnings (8%) as women (3%). Women's greater likelihood of poverty is indicated by the higher percentage receiving Supplementary Pension, 15% compared with 7% of men.

The significance of the gender differences in source of income becomes clearer when the distribution of weekly income amounts from different sources for elderly women and men is plotted, as in Figure 5.2. Three pairs of 'box-and-whisker' plots for state benefits, total income excluding non-state pensions, and total income are shown. The distribution of income from all state benefits (first pair of boxplots) is, as one might expect, relatively compressed; the interquartile range is from £38.00 to £43.00 for men and from £23.00 to £40.00 for women. The median income for women, £37.00, is only slightly less than that of men, £40.00. The addition of earnings and interest (second pair of boxplots) has little effect on the spread of incomes, except to raise the top decile for elderly men to £64.00 per week.

However, when non-state pensions are added (third pair of boxplots), a dramatic differentiation of incomes can be seen. There is a substantial spreading of the income distribution for men, while that of women is scarcely altered. The effect has been to raise the median income of elderly men from £41.00 to £55.00 per week, to raise the upper quartile limit from £45.00 to £80.00 per week and the top decile from £64.00 to £121.00 per week. Thus non-state pensions are the major source of the gender differences in income shown in Figure 5.1.

In order to assess the extent to which women's disadvantage in non-state pension income is related to the gendered labour market and to their past contributions to the domestic economy, receipt and amount of non-state pension is analysed by gender, marital status and occupational class. Comparison of non-state pension income between never-married (i.e. single) elderly women and men provides a measure of the effect of gender alone, while comparison between marital statuses for each sex indicates the effect of position in the domestic economy.

Gender Differences in Non-state Pension Income

Table 5.2 shows the gender difference in receipt of non-state pension income in later life. But the amount of pension received is as relevant as likelihood of receipt: among all elderly people, including those who have no non-state pension income, 50% of men, but only 20% of women, receive more than £5.00 per week, while 26% of men and only 7% of women receive over £25.00 per week. A convenient summary measure which we shall use for comparison of women's and men's pension income in each marital status and occupational class is the amount above which 25% of pension incomes lie (referred to as the upper quartile limit).

Table 5.2 Percentage of elderly people receiving non-state pension by gender and marital status.

Marital Status	*Men* %	*Men* N=	*Women* %	*Women* N=	*All* %	*All* N=
Married*	67	(2126)	12	(1621)	43	(3747)
Widowed	60	(537)	34	(2180)	39	(2717)
Div/Sep	44	(72)	28	(98)	35	(170)
Single**	46	(194)	47	(441)	47	(635)
Total	*64*	*2929*	*27*	*4340*	*42*	*7269*

* Married or cohabiting
** Never married

Source: General Household Survey 1985/86 (own analysis)

The rates of non-state pension receipt by gender and marital status are shown graphically in Figure 5.3.

Elderly married men are most likely to receive a pension and divorced, separated or single men are least likely to, with widowers being intermedi-

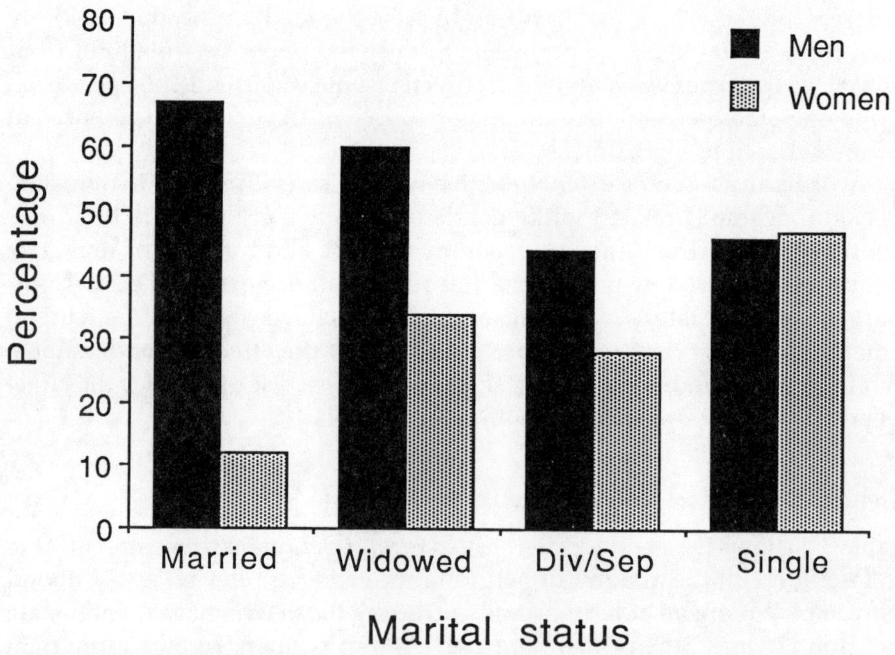

Source: General Household Survey 1985/86 (own analysis)

Figure 5.3: Percentage of elderly people receiving non-state pension by gender and marital status

ate. For elderly women this pattern is almost reversed, as in a mirror image. Thus married women, with the greatest attachment to the domestic role, are least likely to receive a pension, and single women are most likely to. An equal proportion of single men and women receive non-state pensions, 46%.

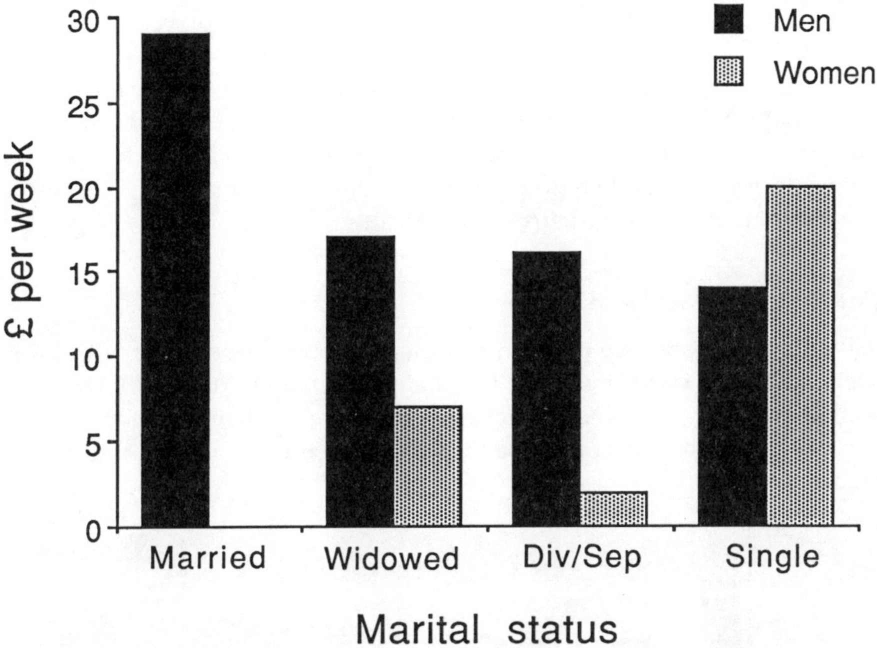

Source: General Household Survey 1985/86 (own analysis)

Figure 5.4: Non-state pension income of elderly people

The upper quartile income limits shown in Figure 5.4 repeat the pattern of relative advantage. For elderly men, pension income increases with attachment to the domestic unit, which suggests that marriage enhances men's pension-earning capacity, but for elderly women the order is reversed.

Widows obtain less pension income than single women, reflecting, as for married women, the constraints of marriage and probably of childrearing on their lifetime earning capacity. They do, however, as a group, have a higher pension income than married or divorced and separated women.

Divorced and separated women are midway between married and single women in likelihood of pension receipt, but their upper quartile pension income is, like that of married women, very low. Through their past domestic position they share with married women and widows the lack of their own non-state pension income, but they have no possibility of currently sharing, or later 'inheriting' a husband's pension.

For single women the upper quartile income limit is actually higher than for single men. A quarter of single elderly women have non-state pension incomes over £20.00 while the same proportion of single men have incomes over £14.00 per week. This last result suggests that gender alone does not fully explain the overall disadvantage of women in non-state pension income. It is, however, possible that single women's advantage may not persist across all socio-economic groups, and this will be explored in the final section.

To summarize, the gendered nature of the domestic economy has resulted in marriage being an advantage for elderly men, at least in terms of acquisition of non-state pension income, and a liability for elderly women. The domestic roles undertaken by women seem to be more important than gender *per se* in limiting their pension income.

The Effect of Class and Gender

Advantage in non-state pension income is strongly associated with higher socio-economic status based on last main occupation, for elderly women as well as men (Figure 5.5). The gender difference holds in each of the seven occupational classes (see Appendix for grouping of socio-economic categories).

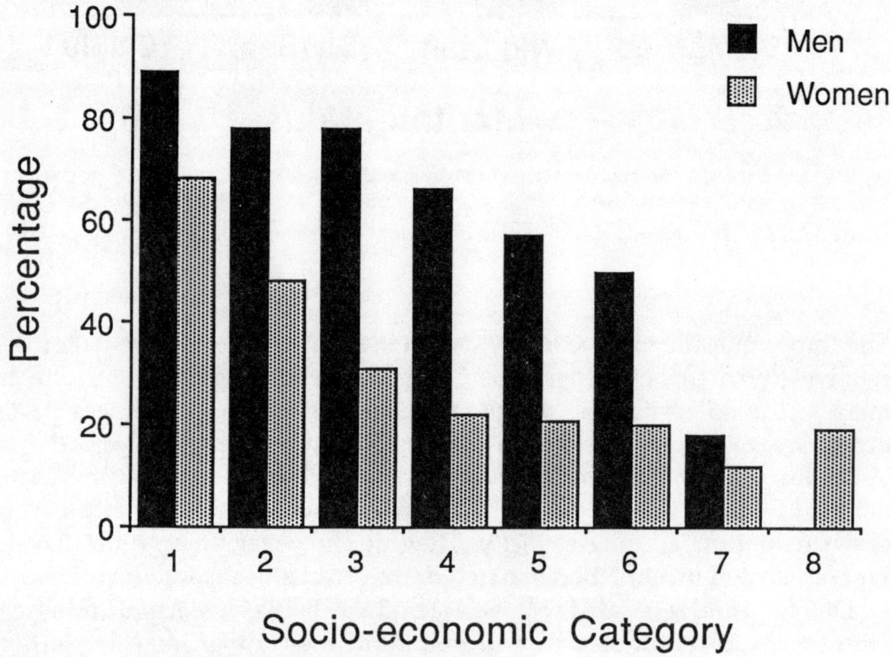

Source: General Household Survey 1985/86 (own analysis)

Figure 5.5: Percentage of elderly people receiving non-state pension by gender and socio-economic category

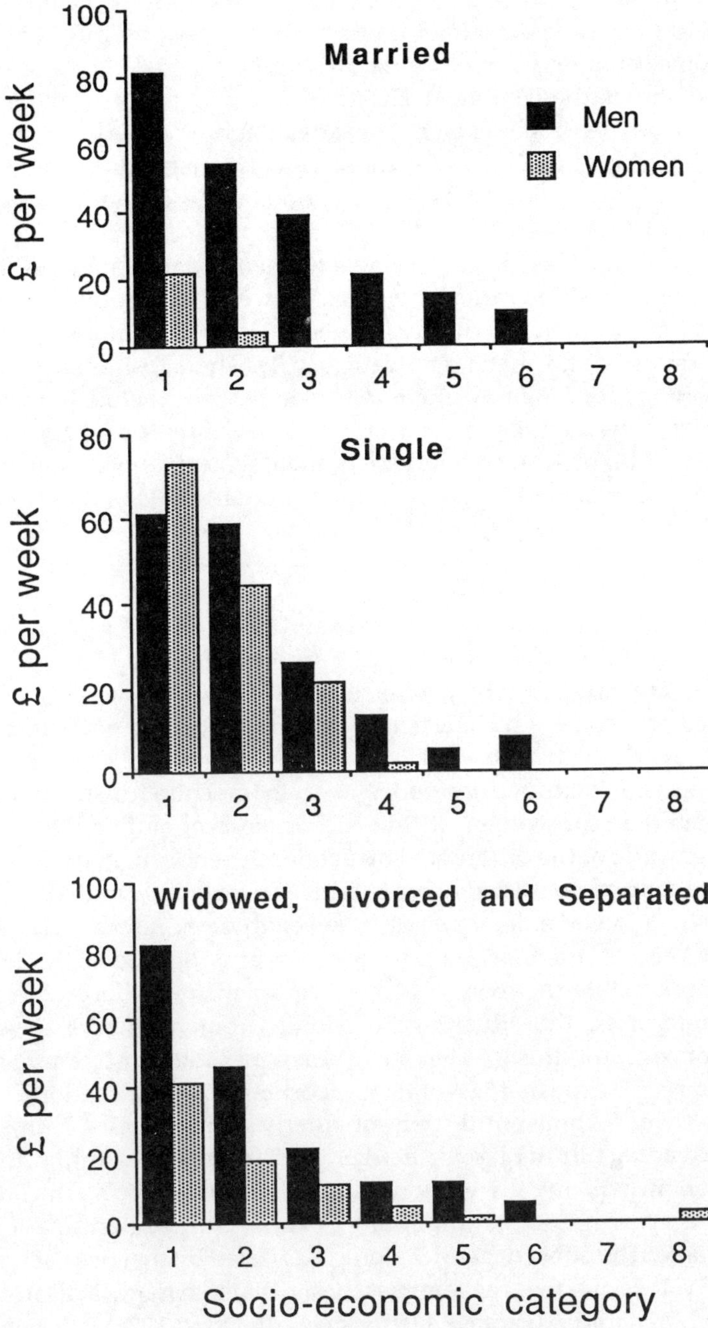

Source: General Household Survey 1985/86 (own analysis)

Figure 5.6: Non state-pension income of elderly people

To find out how sexual divisions in the labour market influence non-state pension receipt, it is necessary to examine occupation-based differences in pension income separately for each marital status.

Figure 5.6 shows the combined effects of last occupation, gender and marital status on pension income. The advantage of elderly men over women persists across all classes for those who are married or previously married, but for single elderly people, previous socio-economic position appears to interact with gender.

Comparison of pension income of single women and men suggested that gender *per se* did not disadvantage women. However, controlling for class shows that single women are disadvantaged relative to men in all classes except professionals and managers (category 1). The substantial pension income advantage for single women over married or previously married women occurs only for those who were in non-manual occupations. All elderly women who previously worked in manual occupations have negligible non-state pensions, irrespective of their marital status.

Discussion

These analyses demonstrate that the substantial inequalities of personal income amongst the sample of over 7000 respondents over 65 in the 1985 and 1986 GHS are structured by gender, marital status and class.

The source of income which decisively differentiates women's incomes from men's, and which also contributes most to inequality of income amongst men, is non-state pensions. Income from this source is substantially higher for men than for women, within each socio-economic group. However, the magnitude of the differential by gender depends on marital status, being greatest for married elderly people and least for single, with divorced, separated and widowed elderly people between these extremes. In terms of personal entitlement, the married state for men is associated with highest pension income, while the reverse is the case for women. Controlling for socio-economic class, the advantage of single women relative to other women is not constant. It is greatest for women previously in non-manual occupations and disappears for women in working class occupations.

Thus the lower income entitlement of elderly women arises both from gender disadvantage in the labour market, and from their position in the domestic economy during the working life. These have effects which continue into old age, and are as important as class in the determination of personal income. The effect of gender alone is dwarfed by that of attachment to domesticity. It seems that the feminist thesis, that marriage is disadvantageous for women and advantageous for men, (Bernard 1976) is borne out in the case of personal income from non-state pensions. We must remember, however, Bernard's observation that, due to the 'marriage gradient' (men tending to marry below their status), the men and women who never marry are not comparable in terms of earning potential. This explains most of the advantage in personal income of single women over single men.

Ageism, and the separation, in mainstream research, of the public world of employment and welfare from the private domain of home and family, has obscured these connections between earlier roles in both the formal and the domestic economy and income in later life. The neglect of domestic 'production', and a narrowly economistic approach which recognises only money transfers as relevant to an 'intergenerational balance sheet', has apparently blinded Johnson and his co-authors (1989) to a dilemma for women, (and for those few men who are 'houseworkers' and carers). Disadvantage in the labour market is most acute for those constrained by the roles of wife and mother, a disadvantage perpetuated into old age through occupation-dependent pension schemes. Thus it is women's contribution to bearing and rearing the next generation of employees, as well as servicing those currently employed, which most seriously handicaps them in ensuring their own pension entitlement. For women (in Britain at least), personal poverty is the price of fertility.

But this is not a purely personal dilemma, as demographers have long been aware; one of the major factors in creating the demographic crisis in industrialised societies described by Johnson and his co-authors is the long-term fall in fertility rates. The problem is therefore a social one. Women have historically been treated as 'a mass army, to be marched in one direction – to the family or the factory, the cradle or the computer' (Wicks 1989) by governments' exhortations, yet they are currently being urged in both directions at once. The traditional family with mother at home to care for children, husband, elderly relatives and neighbours is idealised. It is presented as a convenient panacea against all those trends defined as social problems, and used to justify cuts in public provision. At the same time, the 1990s are heralded as 'the decade of the working woman' (Norman Fowler MP, quoted in Wicks 1989).

Are women to care for kin and ensure the future of society, or should they concentrate on securing their own financial future? In Britain at present these are incompatible objectives for most women. Whether in the future elderly women will suffer long-term poverty depends on whether policies are developed now to enable women to pursue full-time continuous employment while the caring role is collectively shared; or alternatively policies which recognise the value of domestic labour, both during childrearing and in later life, and remunerate it accordingly.

Summary

Our analysis has confirmed that conceptualising elderly people as a homogeneous group in terms of income is very misleading, in view of the magnitude and structure of income inequalities. Non-state pension income is crucial to this structuring, providing a mechanism for the perpetuation of inequalities associated with previous position in both the productive and reproductive economies. As non-state pensions become more common among those retiring in the 1990s, income inequalities among elderly people are likely to increase.

To understand the structure of personal income distribution among elderly people, it is essential to examine gender and marital status, as well as class. The effect of women's unpaid role as houseworkers (indicated by marital status) is more important in explaining their lower personal income in later life than gender *per se*. Only a gender-blind perspective could characterise the relationship between workers and pensioners as conflictual: if there is a conflict of interest, it is not so much between generations as between those who have, during working life, held an advantageous position in both the labour market and the domestic economy – and those who have not.

Acknowledgements

The research on which this paper is based is part of a 2-year project on Community Care and the Elderly funded by the ESRC (Grant No. R000231458). For access to the General Household Survey data for 1985 and 1986, we are indebted to the ESRC Data Archive, University of Essex, and to the University of London Computing Centre. We are grateful to the Office of Population Censuses and Surveys for permission to use the GHS data.

References

Arber, S. (1989) Class and the Elderly, *Social Studies Review* 4 (3) 90–95.

Bernard, J. (1976) *The Future of Marriage,* Harmondsworth: Penguin.

Binstock, R. (1984) Reframing the Agenda of Policies on Aging. In Minkler, M. and Estes, C. (eds) *Readings in the Political Economy of Aging,* New York: Baywood.

Bradshaw, J. and O'Higgins, M. (1984) *Equity, Income Inequality and the Life Cycle; an Analysis for 1971, 1976 and 1982,* University of York, mimeo.

Caplow, T. (1954) *The Sociology of Work.* New York: McGraw-Hill.

Dex, S. (1985) *The Sexual Division of Work.* Brighton: Wheatsheaf Books.

Dex, S. and Phillipson, C. (1986) Social Policy and the Older Worker'. In Phillipson, C. and Walker, A. (eds) *Ageing and Social Policy: a Critical Assessment,* Aldershot: Gower.

Evandrou, M. and Victor, C. (1989) Differentiation in Later Life: Social Class and Housing Tenure Cleavages. In Bytheway, B., et al (eds) *Becoming and Being Old: Sociological Approaches to Later Life.* London: Sage.

Evans, J. (1983) *Marriages and Money: Forms of Financial Arrangement within the Family,* mimeo. University of Surrey Sociology Department.

Edwards, M. (1981) *Financial Arrangements within Families.* Canberra: National Women's Advisory Council.

Fries, J. (1980) Ageing, Natural Death and the Compression of Morbidity, *New England Journal of Medicine* 303 (3) 130.

Glendinning, C. and Millar, J. (1987) Invisible Women, Invisible Poverty. In Glendinning, C. and Millar, J. (eds) *Women and Poverty in Britain.* Brighton: Wheatsheaf.

Gordon, M. (1963) Income Security Programs and the Propensity to Retire. In R. Williams, T. Clark, and W. Donahue (eds), *Processes of Aging,* New York: Atherton Press.

Greene, V. (1989) Editorial, *The Gerontologist* 29 (6) 273–4.

Graham, H. (1987) Women's Poverty and Caring. In Glendinning, C. and Millar, J. (eds), (op. cit.).

Groves, D. (1987) Occupational Pension Provision and Women's Poverty in Old Age'. In Glendinning, C. and Millar, J. (eds), (op. cit.).

Hakim, C. (1979) *Occupational Segregation, Research Paper no. 9.* London: Department of Employment.

Hedstrom, P. and Ringen, S. (1987) *Age and Income in Contemporary Society,* Stockholm: Swedish Institute for Social Research.

Johnson, P., Conrad, C. and Thomson, D. (eds) (1989) *Workers Versus Pensioners: Intergenerational Conflict in an Ageing World,* Manchester University Press.

Johnson, P. (1989) The Structured Dependency of the Elderly: a Critical Note. In Jefferys, M. (ed) *Growing Old in the Twentieth Century.* London: Routledge.

Joshi, H. (1987) The Cost of Caring. In Glendinning, C. and Millar, J. (eds) (op.cit.)

Klein, V. (1965) *Britain's Married Women Workers.* London: Routledge and Kegan Paul.

Labour Research Department (1988) *The LRD Guide to Pensions Bargaining.* London: LRD Publications.

Laslett, P. (1987) The Emergence of the Third Age, *Ageing and Society* (7) 133–160.

Longman, P. (1987) *Born to Pay: the New Politics of Aging in America.* Boston: Houghton Mifflin.

Martin, J. and Roberts, C. (1984) *Women and Employment: a Lifetime Perspective.* London: HMSO.

Mason, J. (1987) A Bed of Roses? Women, Marriage and Inequality in Later Life. In P. Allatt, T. Keil, A. Bryman and B. Bytheway, *Women and the Life Cycle.* Basingstoke: Macmillan.

Millar, J. and Glendinning, C. (1989) Gender and Poverty, *Journal of Social Policy* 18 (3) 363–81.

Minkler, M. (1984) Introduction. In Minkler, M. and Estes, C. (eds) *Readings in the Political Economy of Aging.* New York: Baywood.

Oakley, A. (1974) *The Sociology of Housework.* Oxford: Martin Robertson.

Office of Population Censuses and Surveys (1988) *General Household Survey 1985.* London: HMSO.

Office of Population Censuses and Surveys (1989) *General Household Survey 1986*. London: HMSO.

Pahl, J. (1980) Patterns of Money Management within Marriage, *Journal of Social Policy* 9 (3) 313–35.

Pahl, J. (1989) *Money and Marriage*. London: Macmillan Education.

Paterson, G. (1988) The Caring for the Old that Leaves Me Cold, *Sunday Telegraph*, Jan 10th.

Peace, S. (1986) The Forgotten Female: Social Policy and Older Women. In Phillipson, C. and Walker, A. (eds) *Ageing and social policy: a critical assessment*. London: Gower.

Petrie, P. and Logan, P. (1986) *After School and in the Holidays*. Thomas Coram Research Unit, London: Institute of Education.

Phillipson, C. and Walker, A. (eds) (1986) *Ageing and Social Policy: a Critical Assessment*. London: Gower.

Phillipson, C. (1990) *Intergenerational Relations: Conflict or Consensus in the Twenty-first Century*. Paper given at Welfare State Seminar Series, STICERD, LSE, February. (mimeo)

Popay, J. (1989) Poverty and Plenty: Women's Attitudes Towards and Experience of Money across Social Classes. In Graham, H. and Popay, J. *Women and Poverty: Exploring the Research and Policy Agenda*, Thomas Coram Research Unit / University of Warwick, London: Institute of Education.

Sen, A. (1984) Rights and Capabilities. In Sen, A. *Resources, Values and Development*. Oxford: Basil Blackwell.

Spiers, B. and Spiers, P. (1990) *The Woman's Guide to the State Pension and Income Tax*. London: Greater London Association for Pre-Retirement.

Townsend, P. (1981) The Structured Dependency of the Elderly: a Creation of Social Policy in the Twentieth Century, *Ageing and Society* 1 (1) 5–28.

Vogler, C. (1989) *Labour Market Change and Patterns of Financial Allocation within Households, Working Paper no. 12*, ESRC.

Walker, A. (1986) Pensions and the Production of Poverty in Old Age. In Phillipson, C. and Walker, A. (op. cit.)

Walker, A. (1987) The Poor Relation: Poverty Among Old Women. In Glendinning, C. and Millar, J. (op. cit.)

Wells, N. and Freer, C. (eds) (1988) *The Ageing Population: Burden or Challenge?* London: Macmillan.

Wicks, M. (1989) Where does the Government think a Woman's Place is?, *The Independent*, January 1st 1989.

Appendix

Grouping Of Socio-economic Categories From OPCS Socio-economic Groups (of Respondents Last Occupation)

Socio-Economic Categories	*Description of Groups Included*	*OPCS SEGs **
1	Professionals (employees and self-employed) Managers (large)	1.2,3,4
2	Intermediate non-manual,foremen and ancillary, Managers (small)	2.2,5
3	Junior non-manual	6
4	Manual workers (skilled), foremen and supervisory	8,9
5	Personal service, Semi-skilled manual and agricultural workers	7,10,15
6	Unskilled manual workers	11
7	Employers (large and small, including farmers) Own-account workers (farmers and non-professionals)	1.1,2.1,12,13,14
8	Never worked	
Excluded	Armed forces, full-time students, No answer, or inadequate description	16,17

*OPCS (1980) Classification of Occupations, 1980, Appendix C, London: HMSO

CHAPTER 6

Groupwork and Professional Attitudes to Older Age

Simon Biggs

Many writers have discussed an ambivalence that the helping professions adopt toward the older person as a user of services (Norman 1987, Hildebrand 1982, Bender 1984, Phillipson and Strang 1986). Whilst bearing little relation to the expressed experience of older people themselves (Victor 1987, Biggs 1989), such views are held in common with the everyday construction of older age in the general population (Gubrium and Wallace 1990). Prejudice against older people, at least in western industrial society, begins at an early age and has been found in the verbal and non-verbal behaviour of six-year-old children (Isaacs and Bearison 1986).

In social work Goldberg et al (1970) have noted the 'stoic acceptance' shown toward the circumstances of older service users, which was thought to be typical and unamenable to change. Rowlings (1987) indicates a widespread pessimism in professional thinking about the value of work with older clients, whilst Jones (1987) reports old age as seen as a time of despair, futility and dependency. Heycox (1989) has shown that these attitudes often translate into self-imposed limitations in work with elders, inaction and a lack of creative responding to problems as they arise. Similar attitudes have been discovered in a review of nursing care (Chandler *et al* 1986), in the views of home help organisers (Leslie and Fowell 1988), and physical therapists (Barta Kivek *et al* 1986).

Professional education is, unsurprisingly given the above, also prone to bias. Phillipson and Strang's (1986) survey of training for helping professionals showed that, in spite of the fact that both training and experience was disproportionately weighted towards children and families, 'it was characteristic for professionals to assume that they were in touch with both the emotional and material needs of their (aged) clients, and that they possessed adequate "theoretical" knowledge about old age'. I have argued elsewhere (Biggs 1989, 1990) that, in the absence of information or direct experience of older age, younger workers fill this 'gap' with the predominantly negative stereotypes surrounding them in their wider society. A lack of understanding that the existential dilemmas and life tasks of older age differ from those of helpers, who will themselves be struggling with everyday problems appropriate to their own stages of life, means that the latter are used to evaluate and even replace the expressed requirements of the older person.

In any encounter between two people, and the relationship between a professional helper and a service user is no exception, it is important not only to take into account the effect one has on the other, but also the effect the other has on oneself. These effects are not exclusively conscious, and in the language of the psychotherapies are referred to as transference and counter-transference respectively. The primary consideration here is that of counter-transference, namely the effect that an older person has on the younger worker, both in terms of the overt associations that arise and ones that are not necessarily immediately available to consciousness. The latter may be made available through supervision and group experience, and their effects on the behaviour of the worker open to reflection and change.

These attitudes do not, however, spring exclusively from the relationship between two people. They are shaped by the social circumstances that both parties find themselves in and the background of folk images and social stereotypes that have been attributed to the social categories that participants belong to. This paper examines the special effects of transference and counter-transference with older age, and goes on to consider the phenomenon of social stereotyping before looking in more detail at two groupwork approaches that have used insights from both traditions.

Transference and Counter-transference

Knight (1986) has defined transference and counter-transference in the following manner:

> Transference is the development of a relationship with the therapist by the client that is not based on the reality of the therapeutic relationship or on the therapist's real characteristics as a human-being. Similarly, counter-transference represents the therapists perception of a relationship with the client that is not based on the reality of the relationship or the clients actual characteristics. (p.131)

Whether mis-perceptions that arise are always a hindrance to real communication that should be eliminated, or are a form of information that can be used on the road to a deeper understanding of human relationships has been a matter of debate from the earliest exploration of the phenomenon. Freud took the former view, whereas Jung preferred a more flexible interactive approach (Jacoby 1984).

What has become clear more recently is that this exchange of not necessarily conscious attitudes takes on a particular form in the case of how the younger therapist uses associations about older age (a development not enhanced by Freud's own unhelpful observation that people over the age of 40 'are no longer educable' (Freud 1904). Knight (1986) has identified the following factors that influence an older person's view of the young helper. The helper may be responded to as their child, grandchild, parent or spouse at a younger age. The traditional helper-helped relationships is to some extent reversed by these associations (Rechtschaffen 1959) which may both unnerve and threaten the helper. As part of this process, the helper in work with older people 'may confront current issues in her or his own life and may also confront future issues that are now only fearful fantasies'. The Committee on Aging of the Group for the Advancement of Psychiatry (1971) has identified a number of negative reactions that helping staff might have to work through with elders. Fears of personal ageing, conflict with ones own parental figures, belief in the older persons inability to change, nearness to death and thus a misallocation of resources, and finally the contemptuous attitude of colleagues, all contribute to distance helpers from the older service user.

The effects of such negative attitudes, as a contributing factor to a reduced service to older people have been well documented in the study of residential care (Wilkin and Hughes 1987, Booth *et al* 1990) and will not be elaborated here. Several observers also note the deleterious effects on decisions about personal counselling (Hildebrand 1982, Pfieffer 1971). The helper may respond by avoidance, by not providing services, speeding up the process of helping and by suggesting physical rather than directly interpersonal forms of intervention. In some cases, workers may succumb to an alternative omnipotent response, a 'messiah complex' (Sprung 1989) or 'manna personality' (Fordham 1953) whereby the requirements of the older person are swamped by the workers' need to 'do something' or do good. Both types of personal response, avoidance and omnipotence may be seen, however, to feed the workers own priorities and re-establishment of positional power rather than address the reality of the older person's life situation.

Ageism

A parallel strand of investigation into relationships between older and younger people arises from the study of Ageism. In the British context, much of this work has its roots in the analysis of structural inequality such as pensionable age and the unequal distribution of resources to older people in need, as compared to other sectors of this population (Townsend 1986, Phillipson 1982, Walker 1986). Other writers have drawn parallels between ageism and other oppressions such as sexism and racism (Itzin 1986, Butler 1987). Levin and Levin (1980) have proposed that elders constitute a minority group in themselves, although this view has been disputed (Hopkins 1980, Bytheway and Johnson 1990). Shonfield (1982) has suggested that there is enough contradictory evidence to invalidate a distinctive constellation of prejudice, called ageism. Whether or not ageism is a construct of over-enthusiastic gerontology or not, several writers have shown that older age is a significant contributing factor to the experience of oppression by women

(Finch and Groves 1985, Le Riche and Rowlings 1990) and black people (Patel 1990, Ahmed 1988). 'It is facile' state Bytheway and Johnson (1990) 'to suppose that (older people) might associate with one social group to the exclusion of others, that their deprivation is due to one characteristic rather than to a complex pattern of circumstances and that they are untouched, for example, by the ageism within the women's movement, the sexism within black organisations and the racism within pensioner organisations'.

The particular quality that older age brings in relation to younger others, at this point in time, would seem to the writer to centre on passive omission, and thus exclusion. This has been expressed by Comfort (1977) as 'the notion that people cease to be people, cease to be the same people or become people of a distinct and inferior kind, by virtue of having lived a specified number of years'.

This notion helps to explain how work with older people so easily falls prey to a preoccupation with the psychological priorities and conflicts of younger people as described in the preceding section of this paper.

Attitudes to Older Age: Summary

So far, two streams of analysis, the psychological and the political, have been examined in order to throw light on relations between younger workers and older service users. The former has provided information on the 'fine-tuning' of interpersonal relationships and the inner world of the helper. The latter increases awareness of how structural inequality requires a focus on power as a determining factor in the process of inter-group relations.

Groupwork

It is now time to examine the particular value of groupwork as a means of raising issues of power in an interpersonal context. For the purposes of this paper, groupwork will refer to the time limited experiences of between approximately five and eighteen people who come together to reflect in a focused way on a defined issue. Both the content and process of the group can be used to deepen understanding. That is to say, exercises that the group undertakes to generate memories, issues and activities plus observations on how participants combine and respond to this material, would be studied. First, some of the qualities of work in groups will be summarised. Two approaches, that of 'Confronting Ageing' (Biggs 1989) and 'Ageism Awareness Training' (Itzin 1986) will be compared and contrasted. Finally, some conclusions will be drawn on training for professional helpers.

Why Groupwork?

When compared to individual tuition or formal training, working in small groups has certain advantages for the training of helping professionals.

These advantages are particularly important when examining attitudes and social stereotypes. Four specific advantages can be identified.

First, participants are exposed to the different experiences of group members. This is valuable as most people have an implicit guiding hypothesis that their own experience of family life, attitudes to old age and older people are somehow 'the norm' and that others hold the same opinion. By comparing family experiences and attitudes of differently aged persons the diversity of 'normal' experience can be explored. In cases where issues are taboo or are rarely allowed an arena for discussion (such as fears of personal ageing) the discovery that some attitudes and reservations are commonly held can also be liberating.

Second, the possibility of sharing collective experience and common stereotypes in relative anonymity (for example, by writing them down oneself and then pooling unnamed responses via the group leader), can combine the advantages of personal reflection with the unattributed views of others. Participants can adopt roles that best suit their own personal style, whilst learning about the style of others. As groups are essentially social phenomena, the possibility of identifying and comparing stereotypes is that much easier.

Third, it is possible to observe and reflect upon the behaviour of others and the process of examining issues itself. This is a valuable tool in preparing participants for life in the world outside the group where they will need to understand the reactions of others to open discussion of older age and its impact.

Finally, the group allows the formation of a collective plan which a team, or collection of disparate individuals can use as a point of reference and support in addressing change in existing service delivery systems.

An experienced groupworker may also divide participants into subgroups with professional membership, race, gender or age in common to compare the different experiences that such perspectives bring with them. Essentially, groupwork engages with a subtext that attitudes are socially constructed and that solutions involve interdependency.

Confronting Ageing and the Negative Personal Future

I have argued elsewhere, in an attempt to explain the reasoning behind a number of groupwork exercises (Biggs 1990), that younger workers find themselves in a unique position with regard to a disadvantaged and therefore partial picture of older people, which holds implications for education and training. These are itemised below and have implications for successful education and training.

1. Younger helpers have no direct experience of old age, and limited exposure to elders.

2. In the absence of meaningful contact, rigid stereotypes and images of old age can fill this vacuum.
3. Many helpers expect their own old age to be a negative experience.
4. The life-tasks and projects of younger and older adults differ in content and in ascribed social value.
5. The above factors can lead to avoidance or replacement of elders' needs in line with the age-related preoccupations of the helper.
6. In some cases helpers may unreflectively abuse a sense of personal power arising from work with elders.

> 'It is not just that workers mix with a disadvantaged group of old people and take this to represent the whole population, although this is important. The 'taking to be the whole'... makes it extremely difficult to confront a personally acceptable view of their own ageing' (Biggs 1989, p.51).

This personal future, often seen as negative and inevitable, can lead workers to eschew contact with situations that provoke recognition of a presumed state of affairs awaiting them as well. Beneath this first response the groupworker may find a number of complex psychological factors that depend on personal experience and the work environment where elders are primarily encountered. Using constructs originally arising from Jungian psychology (Jung 1933) it is possible to hypothesise intra-psychic mechanisms that contribute to the particular imbalance of power that arises at the point where those who deliver services meet those who need them.

Working Life and Hidden Parts of the Self

Working life requires a limited personal development. Jung (1933) has proposed that the 'first half of life', which roughly corresponds to that spent at work, is characterised by individualism, external achievement, a 'diminution of the personality' that suppresses other parts of the self by pushing them into the unconscious. This is not to say that this suppressed 'shadow side' fails to make itself felt, especially when one comes in contact with others whose characteristics correspond to these unacknowledged parts which can then be projected onto them.

The life tasks of older age, on the other hand, have been associated with integrating the whole self, thereby giving reign to parts that have previously been inconvenient or actively repressed. This process, labelled 'individuation' by Jung, involves withdrawing projections from others as a route to maintaining self-esteem. Such processes are supported by Guttman's (1988) observations that people change to a more 'balanced' personality in older life, particularly with respect to men taking on more 'feminized' roles and vice versa. As part of this re-adjustment in the 'second half of life', the older person uses experience to assist those 'who are still developing' thereby indirectly influencing the working or family world.

If, as this argument suggests, repression of parts of the personality is related to age and associated life tasks, then it is reasonable to conclude that contact with elders presents an opportunity for hidden and contextually inconvenient parts of the helper's own self to be tickled into consciousness. Moreover, as the elder may desire that their own experience be validated and even be helpful to the younger worker, the latter's power enshrined in being the active 'helper' is also implicitly threatened.

In situations where the rest of a professional's work takes place with younger people or peers, it is relatively easy for an elder's attempts to express their own age-appropriate tasks to be seen as inappropriate. In the sense that when working with peers, life tasks are held in common and therefore taken for granted as part of the 'common sense' (Schutz 1983) of expected interactions whilst different, 'older' goals disrupt this hitherto invisible assumed reality. In the case of work with younger users, the worker has some experience of life to draw on, and it is possible that the relationship, in age-appropriate terms, is more easily defined.

Unconscious Images of Elders

A second contribution from Jungian psychology concerns the content of this 'shadow side'. It is striking, given the predominantly negative conscious awareness of older age, to encounter the potentially positive image that appears in dreams. Here, the 'Wise Elder' often appears as a bringer of change, a 'transitional' figure who evidences the possibility of moving beyond ones current circumstances, by highlighting the opposite of what is consciously apparent. Given the tendency of the shadow self to contain the opposite, it is perhaps itself an indication of the direction of attitudes to ageing that this unconscious image of elders is both positive and transforming, rather than negative and passive.

However, any such challenge from the unconscious, provoked either by contact with real older people or dissatisfaction with a youthful life stage, can either be embraced or rejected in daily life. Although an individual is eventually 'capable of taking the projected transference of what they will become,... at first the content of the projection may take the form of one who is preventing the same initiative' (Samuels, Shorter and Plant 1986). In other words, 'Individuals or groups who trigger a potentially transforming image may be experienced negatively and give rise to unpleasant feelings because the person experiencing intra-psychic associations sees these qualities as an impediment to the state he or she is presently in. One thus becomes the bringer of ambivalent news' (Biggs 1989). Now, if the situation where younger and older people meet is sufficiently formal, distanced, and unbalanced in terms of power, it is unlikely that personal contact will counteract internal stereotypes or defences. Avoiding such alienating environments would be a necessary prerequisite for a more flexible and humanised relationship both between participants and within their intra psychic worlds. Unfortunately, this is often resisted in practice.

The temptation to use institutional defences (Menzies 1970) to protect oneself from threats to the established psychic order in part explains how, in Wilkin and Hughes (1987) words, 'people who have spent a lifetime of independence find themselves often unwillingly having to live with others and become dependent for many of the requirement of life'. Control of the elder becomes part and parcel of a workers defences against personal old age. It is argued then, that the supposed negative future, lopsided development in working life and potentially threatening internal images of old age, contribute to an omission of expressed and age-appropriate goals of an older person, in favour of ones which better fit, or ones made sense of in terms of working helpers' own age-related tasks. Such a substitution is enhanced by the degraded status of older people who are no longer themselves working (and thus not seen as 'productive') and are more often asking for support rather than being in control of resources themselves.

The Confronting Ageing Approach

The Confronting Ageing Approach (CAA) attempts to replace personal anticipations of a negative future by challenging a monolithic definition of age (by considering how old one feels, how old one would like to be, chronological age, feelings at age 75, etc) and distinguishing between stereotypes of 'Old People' and perceptions of an older person who is well known. The limited contact between age-cohorts is also challenged.

CAA moves from personal experience of age and ageing, through stereotypes, to an examination of the use and abuse of power in interpersonal relationships across ages in the workplace. Finally, what group members would require in their own old age is linked to empowerment of elder service users and a critical examination of existing service delivery systems. Links are made at this point between the experience of older people and that of other disadvantaged groups who use services. A typical combination of group-work exercises has been reproduced in Table 6.1 and a more detailed exposition of work using the approach can be found in Biggs (1990).

Ageism Awareness Training

Ageism Awareness Training (AAT, Itzin 1986) has its roots in the co-counselling movement. It sees prejudice against older people as part of a wider problem of 'adultism', i.e. the abuse of power by those in the middle or adult years against children and elders.

Observations that 'Adults have rights and privileges which are denied to young people and older people' leads Itzin to examine individual socialisation as a means of making links between group members' own experience

Table 6.1 Groupwork Exercises

	Title	*Activity*	*Function*
Session 1	General and personal (3.1) How old? (1.1)	Compare association to phrase 'Old People' with 'Older person known personally'. Personal age categories.	To explore nature and extent of stereotypes.
Session 2	Generations (2.1) Mass media (3.2) Knowledge (4.1)	Note contact with persons of different ages over a defined time period. Consider where information comes from.	Degree and context of actual contact. Sources of information.
Session 3	When I am old (1.3) Different perspectives (4.5)	Guided fantasy to own old age. Role play / psychodrama for Old person, Helper, or Carer.	To explore degrees of entouchedness, power, communication patterns and collusive alliances.
Session 4	Your Own 'Carer' (3.5) Consumer Choice (4.9)	What participants want in old age. Planning service systems and consumer involvement.	Enlightened self interest. Application to work-context.

Reproduced from Biggs (1990) Ageism and Confronting Ageing: experential groupwork to examine attitudes to older age. Journal of Social Work Practice (4.2) 49–65.
* Numbers in brackets refer to designated exercises from 'Confronting Ageing',

of oppression during childhood with that of the dis-empowered state of older age. The key to personal liberation from ageist or adultist behaviour and attitudes is to encounter again the 'internalised oppression' engendered during childhood by adultist others. Once the experience of personal invalidation has been rediscovered, it is possible for group members to 'reclaim the power that was diminished or denied', an experience that is then used to change 'relationships with one or more old people', and 'things they can do' at work.

In practical terms, AAT poses a number of questions for the group to consider, which are introduced in order by a facilitator (see Table 6.2). The questions begin at the age participants are now, then move on to a consideration of personal childhood and relations with adults. Attitudes toward older people and personal ageing follow. The questions conclude by examining the personal decision to change relationships with known elders and address ageism at work.

Comparing AAT and CAA

There are many parallels between the two methods. Both see prejudice against older people as a stereotype with personal and structural implica-

Table 6.2. Questions from Ageism Awareness Training (Itzin 1986)

Starting with the age we are

1. How old are you?
2. What is good about being the age you are now?

Working on adultism

3. What did you most enjoy about being a child?
4. What did you most hate about being a child?
5. How did you manage, as a child, to 'outwit' the adults and to maintain your integrity?
6. What would you like to say now, with what you know from your position as an adult, to the little 'you' then?

Working on ageism

7. What do you like about old people?
8. Tell us about an old person you have been close to and what you have liked about them?
9. What can't you stand about older people?
10. What is your greatest fear about growing old (or older) or being old?
11. How should it be, for you, when you are old?
12. What would you say to your older 'future self' from where you stand now?
13. If there were no adultism or ageism, if you were confident and without fear, how would your relations with old people be different now?

Deciding to change

14. What specific changes in a relationship with one or more old people would you like to make from this point on?
15. What is one thing you are going to do to change ageist practices in your workplace and the structures of ageism in your profession or society?

tions which result in an inability to work humanly with elders. Both also rely on enlightened self-interest as a bridge between younger worker and older consumer in the absence of empathic experience of older age itself, albeit in different ways. AAT is perhaps more directive, the questions leading participants to certain conclusions, whereas CAA relies on the juxtaposition of selected group exercises to encourage members to draw their own conclusions.

There are also marked differences. CAA relies on self-interest by emphasising the participants future role as a service user and the liberating effects of relativity, of 'freeing-up' evaluation of their future old age. By contrast AAT attempts to use the liberating power of a re-evaluation of childhood experience in the service of identification with older people. Interpersonal inequality is seen, in CAA, as primarily focused on power relations in the provision of services, between users and professional helpers, whereas AAT focuses on inequality based on age as the determining factor. This is not to say that each exclusively refers to a single causal factor. CAA, with its underlying analysis of the invalidation and replacement of elders' existential age-related priorities by those of the younger professional, and AAT with its guiding principle of oppression within the whole of society both take account of different levels of inequality in human relationships. However, the differences noted above lead to a significant parting of the ways over the aims and function of work with attitudes.

By using 'adultism' as a unifying concept, AAT comes to certain conclusions that could be seen as problematic. First, it is unclear whether children's and older people's oppression are similar, other than in the abstract experience of unfairness engendered in the adult participant. The tendency to define elders as 'not adult' that the analysis implies, plus the all-too-close equivalence of elders and children presents difficulties. If the adult group member is encouraged to use his or her intouchedness with childhood as the basis of personal liberation in such a direct manner, how far does this encourage alienation from the reality of their everyday adult age, and from other adult groups, such as fellow workers, or marginalised or disadvantaged adults who may have other experiences in common with older people? Psychologically speaking it is tempting to locate those 'bad' parts in an outside 'adult' world, especially when the questions only refer to the 'goodness' of participants themselves. Unfortunately, Kinnon (1988) has found that similar splitting of attitudes in related methods such as Racism Awareness Training can actually lead to abstention when participants feel helpless or unwilling to change contaminating external circumstances. Similarly, it is not at all clear that the power gained from casting off one's own childhood oppression will be used in the service of older people. Given the unequal institutional context in which contact often takes place, it is easy for this power to be used in an egocentric manner (Fordham 1953, Biggs 1989, Sprung 1989) which, whilst reinforcing the professional's feeling of effectiveness, has little to do with the users' requirements. These problems are not helped by AATs reliance on personal agency as the almost exclusive means of changing relationships and institutional oppression.

CAA is also open to criticism. First, by frequently referring back to the service sector as the locus of interaction, it is unclear how far methods are applicable to other contexts, such as power within families. Also, although it refers to the common experience of oppression between groups that have been marginalised by service systems, CAA fails to pay attention to how links can be made between these groups and the interaction of oppressions within them. As the opening sentence of *Confronting Ageing* says, 'this is a manual for those who work with older people' (Biggs 1989).

A second problem with CAA is that the analysis of the problem is itself premised on the younger professionals' lack of experience of older age, thus leaving a gap to be filled. Having noted that the existential priorities of those in the younger world of work and raising a family differ from those who have aged beyond these requirements (at least in societally defined terms) it is unclear how enlightened self interest is actually in tune with these unexperienced requirements. The answer is, of course, that one cannot be entirely sure, and that fantasies about ones own needs in older age need to be grounded in open dialogue with elders themselves. CAA may, therefore, best be seen as a method of clearing away the clutter, the roadblocks in everyday thought and feeling that diminish both parties, so that a meaningful exchange can begin.

Conclusions

Given evidence to suggest both an avoidance of work with older people and that the particular psychological needs, even in the most damaged persons (Kitwood 1990) may have a social psychological component, it is important to suggest general guidance on the training of professional helpers that takes these factors into account. I propose the following list, which is by no means exhaustive, to counteract age prejudice and enhance empathic understanding of the experience of older age.

1. Training should directly address the question of a presumed negative future old age amongst intending professionals.
2. Students should be encouraged to examine associations with elders that spring from their own experience and current preoccupations at their particular age-stage.
3. In addition to groupwork, students might look at age-cohorts as a whole rather than selective sections who require services. This may lead on to an examination of cultural structural inequality as well as attributions of worth.
4. Students should be able, as a consequence, to evaluate power relations in the context of giving and receiving services.
5. Contact with older individuals or groups who disconfirm stereotypes and the practice of skills that help articulate the needs that elders express themselves, are required to establish a baseline for forms of other specialist assessment.
6. Where teaching of older age forms part of a wider, life-span approach to human development, or as one part of a general professional education, educators should be aware of the tendency to marginalise older age. Wider stereotypes can be implicitly reinforced by assuming that the topic of older age must necessarily come at the end of a course, when competing pressure such as revision for examination or finding further employment take priority, and reproduce the eclipse of older persons argued throughout this chapter. Placing such teaching at the end of a lifespan course also reinforces notions of inevitable decline, and that theories designed to explain earlier periods of development can be 'carried over' without modification.
7. What is not being argued here is that an examination of attitudes or social inequality can take the place of learning specialist skills or recognizing the actual deficits that accompany older age. Rather the former should be used to critically evaluate and facilitate the appropriate use of such skills

in the pursuit of a more equal relationship between those with skills and those who require their effective use.

References

Ahmed, A. (1988) *Social Services for Black People*. London: National Institute for Social Work.

Barta Kivek, S., Shaver, B. and Blood, M. (1986) Age Bias: Physical Therapists and Older Patients. *Journal of Gerontology* 41 (6) 706–709.

Bender, M. (1984) The Neglect of the Elderly by British Psychologists. *Bulleting of the British Psychological Society* 39, 414–416.

Biggs, S.J. (1989) *Confronting Ageing*. London: CCETSW Publications.

Biggs, S.J. (1989) Professional Helpers and Resistances to Work With Older People. *Ageing and Society* 9, 43–65.

Biggs, S.J. (1990) Ageism and Confronting Ageing: experential groupwork to examine attitudes to older age. *Journal of Social Work Practice* 4 (2) 49–65.

Blakemore, K. (1989) *Does Age Matter? The Case of Old Age in Minority Ethnic Groups*. In Bytheway, B. (ed) Becoming and Being Old. London: Sage.

Booth, T., Bilson, A. and Fowell, I. (1990) Staff Attitudes and Caring Practices in Homes for the Elderly. *British Journal of Social Work* 117–131.

Bytheway, B. and Johnson, J. (1990) On Defining Ageism. *Critical Social Policy* 29, 27–39.

Butler, R.N. (1987) 'Agism'. In Maddox, G.L. *Encyclopaedia of Aging* New York: Springer.

Chandler, J. (1986) Attitudes of Nursing Personnel Towards the Elderly. *The Gerontologist* 26 (4) 551–555.

Comfort, A. (1977) *A Good Age*. London: Mitchell Beasley.

Committee on Ageing (1971) *The Aged and Community Mental Health Group for the Advancement of Psychiatry*. New York.

Finch, J. and Groves, D. (1985) Old Boy – Old Girl. In Brooke, E., and Davis, A. (eds). *Women the Family and Social Work*. London: Tavistock.

Fordham, F. (1953) *An Introduction to Jung's Psychology*. London: Penguin.

Freud, S. (1904) *On Psychotherapy in Collected Papers Vol. 1.* (1956) 258. London: Hogarth Press.

Goldberg, E., Mortimer, A. and Williams, B. (1970) *Helping the Aged*. London: Allen and Unwin.

Guttman, D. (1988) *Reclaimed Powers*. New York: Heineman.

Gubrium, J.F., Wallace, J.B. (1990) Who Theorises Age? *Ageing and Society* 10, 131–149.

Heycox, K. (1989) Self Imposed Limitations: Social Work With the Elderly. *Australian Social Work* 42 (3) 17–23.

Hildebrand, P. (1982) Psychotherapy with Older Patients. *British Journal of Medical Psychology* 555, 19–28.

Hopkins, T. (1980) Understanding Racism, Sexism and Ageism. *Journal of Education Social Work* 16, 63–70.

Isaacs, L.W. and Bearison, D.J. (1986) Development of Childrens Prejudice Against the Aged. *International Journal of Ageing and Human Development* 23 (3) 175–194.

Itzin, K. (1986) Ageism Awareness and Training. Phillipson, C., Bernard, M. and Strang, P. (eds) *Dependency and Interdependency in Old Age*. London: Croom Helm.

Jacoby, M. (1984) *The Analytic Encounter: Transference and Human Relationship*. Toronto: Inner City Books.

Jones, G. (1987) Training Social Workers to Work with Older People. In Glendenning, F. (ed) *Social Work with Older People*. Keele: Beth Johnson Foundation.

Jung, C.G. (1933) *Modern Man in Search of a Soul*. London: Routledge.

Kinnon, U. (1988) Racism Awareness – Who Helps the Client? *Journal of Social Work Practice* 3 (3) 80–91.

Kitwood, T. (1990) The Dialectics of Dementia. *Ageing and Society* 10, 177–196.

Knight, B. (1986) *Psychotherapy with Older Adults*. Beverley Hills: Sage.

Leslie, A. and Fowell, I. (1988) A View of Home Help Service. *Social Services Research* 6, 18–26.

Le Riche, P. and Rowlings, C. (1990) Feminist Groupwork with Older Women. *International Social Work* 33 (2) 121–136.

Levin, J. and Levin, W.C. (1980) *Ageism; Prejudice and Discrimination Against the Elderly*. Belmont, California: Wadsworth.

Norman, A. (1987) *Aspects of Ageism*. London: Centre for Policy on Ageing.

Norman, A. (1986) *Triple Jeopardy: Growing Old in a Second Homeland*. London: Centre for Policy on Ageing.

Patel, N. (1990) *A Race Against Time*. London: Runnymede Trust.

Pfieffer, E. (1971) Psychotherapy with Elderly Patients. Postgraduate Medicine, November 254–258.

Phillipson, C. (1982) *Capitalism and the Construction of Old Age*. London: Macmillan.

Phillipson, C. and Strang, D. (1986) *Training and Education for an Ageing Society*. Working Paper No 3: University of Keele.

Rechtschaffen, A. (1959) Psychotherapy with Geriatric Patients. *Journal of Gerontology* 14, 73–84.

Rowlings, C. (1981) *Society Work with Elderly People*. London: Allen and Unwin.

Samuels, A., Shorter, B. and Plant, F. (1986) *A Critical Dictionary of Jungian Analysis*. London: Free Associations Books.

Schutz, A. (1962) *Collected Papers Vol. 1*. The Hague: Martinis-Nijhoff.

Shonfield, D. (1982) Who is Stereotyping Whom and Why. *The Gerontologist* 22 (3) 267–272.

Sprung, G. (1989) Transferential Issues in Working with Older Adults. *Social Casework* 70 (10) 597–603.

Townsend, P. (1986) Ageism and Social Policy. In Phillipson, C. and Walker, A. (eds) *Ageing and Society Policy*. Aldershot: Gower.

Victor, C. (1987) *Old Age in Modern Society*. London: Croom Helm.

Walker, A. (1986) The Politics of Ageing in Britain. In Phillipson, C., Bernard, M., and Strang, P. (eds) *Dependency and Interdependency in Old Age*. London: Croom Helm.

Wilkin, D. and Hughes, B. (1987) Residential Care of Elderly People. *Ageing and Society* 7, 175–207.

CHAPTER 7

The Geography of Private Residential Care

Christopher W. Smith

Some Historical Background

This chapter is concerned with the availability and distribution of the major categories of residential care for elderly people that are currently available in Great Britain. *Local authority homes* were originally established in 1948 by the National Assistance Act, which transferred responsibility for the elderly from the discarded 'Poor Law' to the local authorities (Mears and Smith 1985, Phillips and Vincent 1986). Such establishments are normally termed 'Part III' homes (in England and Wales) or 'Part IV' homes (in Scotland) since these sections of the Act were responsible for their creation. Under the terms of the Act each local authority had to provide residential accommodation for people who 'by means of age, infirmity or any other circumstances' required care and attention not otherwise available to them. This accommodation was to be managed by the local authority.

By contrast, *private rest homes* have, historically, existed for many years, though often did not care exclusively for elderly people. In recent years large increases have occurred nationally in the numbers of such establishments for reasons derived chiefly from the growing contributions from social security payments to the cost of care. The Registered Homes Act (1984) defines them as: 'any establishment which provides, whether for reward or not, residential accommodation with both board and personal care for persons in need of personal care by reason of age (or) disablement...'. However, rest homes caring for fewer than four people are excluded from the Act and obtaining information on such small homes is accordingly very difficult.

Responsibility for the inspection and registration of rest homes is the task of the local authority social services departments, which are also responsible for environmental health standards, building regulations, planning procedures and maintaining fire precaution standards. It has been noted by Phillips and Vincent (1986) that, previously, residential care homes were regulated under the less stringent Residential Homes Act (1980), which defined the homes principally as nursing homes or hospitals. This definition failed to distinguish between the terms 'care' and 'nursing' and, even since the 1984 Act, the differences are often unclear.

Private nursing homes were defined under Part II of the Registered Homes Act (1984) as 'providing for persons suffering from any sickness, injury or infirmity'. Unlike the private rest homes, they are normally registered by the health authority; in the case of the Nottingham HA a special post as Nurse Adviser for private nursing homes was established in April 1984. Registration of private nursing homes by the health authorities rather than the social services was justified on the basis that nursing care is provided (rest homes do not provide nursing care). Responsibility for the monitoring of staffing qualifications and levels, night supervision, facilities and equipment also lies with the health authorities.

The point has been made by Phillips and Vincent (1986) that the 1984 Act also permits nursing homes to register some beds with both local authority and health authority. This dual registration recognises that an overlap exists between these two private categories, though unfortunately there are no guidelines (or regulations) specifying which type of resident should be catered for in which type of home. Thus Challis (1982), working in Bath, had already noted a large 'grey area' or overlap in categories of people living in private rest and nursing homes at a time before the recent expansion of the private sector.

A practical consideration is the considerable problem of liaison between local authorities and health authorities which can make the dual registration system difficult to operate. Indeed it has been suggested by Carson (1985) and Ross (1985) that, legally, the dual registration system is hardly workable. There is much confusion amongst lay persons and even health care professionals as to the precise differences between the two types of home; one unfortunate consequence of this may be the inappropriate location of an elderly person and consequently inappropriate resulting care.

In 1985 a study commenced within the Nottingham Health Authority (HA) conducted from the Department of Health Care of the Elderly at Nottingham University. Initially the project was intended to monitor local developments within both public and private residential sectors for the elderly population up to 1985; later the study was extended to take account of the rapidly expanding local private sector after 1985. This chapter will describe both pre- and post-1985 developments and discuss the implications of these changes for elderly people both locally and nationally.

Demographic Background

The Nottingham HA is the most southerly and urban of three health authorities within Nottinghamshire (the other two being Central Nottinghamshire and Bassetlaw). In mid-1984 it had a population of 612,800, of which some 86,900 (14.2%) were aged 65 years or over. This compares with a national elderly population which constitutes some 15.1% of the total population of England and Wales (OPCS 1983). Although the Nottingham population is slightly more youthful than the national when the 65+ group alone is examined, projected trends for all Nottinghamshire indicate a dramatic increase in the local retired population – especially including the very elderly – relative to the national population (OPCS 1976, NCC 1982). Thus patterns of residential accommodation for elderly people, and especially the very aged, can be expected to change in response to need up to the turn of the century simply as a result of demographic ageing within the Nottingham area.

Although the large numbers of 'young elderly' today, including those who have taken early retirement, are often active, independent and quite able to live in their own homes, they will naturally form the very elderly (ie those over 75 years) of tomorrow. Moreover, most of these future 'old elderly' will be widowed females who may be unable to live alone in accommodation not designed specifically for elderly people. This trend may be further accentuated by physical illness and the expense of living alone.

Within the Nottingham area an additional peculiarity, probably related to the employment of large numbers of women in the lace and tobacco industries, many of whom migrated to Nottingham earlier in the century, is that even higher than national proportions of elderly women are found locally in the very old age groups. Thus there were 4065 women per 1000 men aged 85 and over in the Nottingham Psychiatric Register Area (NPRA) in 1981. For Great Britain the ratio was 3258:1000. The longer life expectations of these elderly women relative to male life expectations will place a further demand on the existing local residential care system in the future.

Distribution of Residential Care to 1985

Figure 7.1 summarises the distribution of Part III homes, private rest homes and private nursing homes respectively in the Nottingham HA in October 1985 (Notts County Council 1985); boundaries for the social service areas are also marked. At that time, local social service departments normally tried to avoid admitting elderly people to Part III homes (see Figure 7.1A) across the area boundaries, in keeping with the policy of placing elderly people close to their original homes. However, since there were obvious concentrations of homes in certain social service areas, notably Nottingham N, Nottingham NW and Nottingham E, and no homes at all in Nottingham NE and Nottingham W, then the social services often adopted the more flexible system of placing people in homes across these boundaries. Moreover, where a need arose to move people to areas close to relatives and friends, the social services tried to be as sympathetic as possible. When the numbers of places in these homes and the total elderly populations of the different social service areas were considered, the overall provision of places at that time can be seen to be very uneven (Table 7.1).

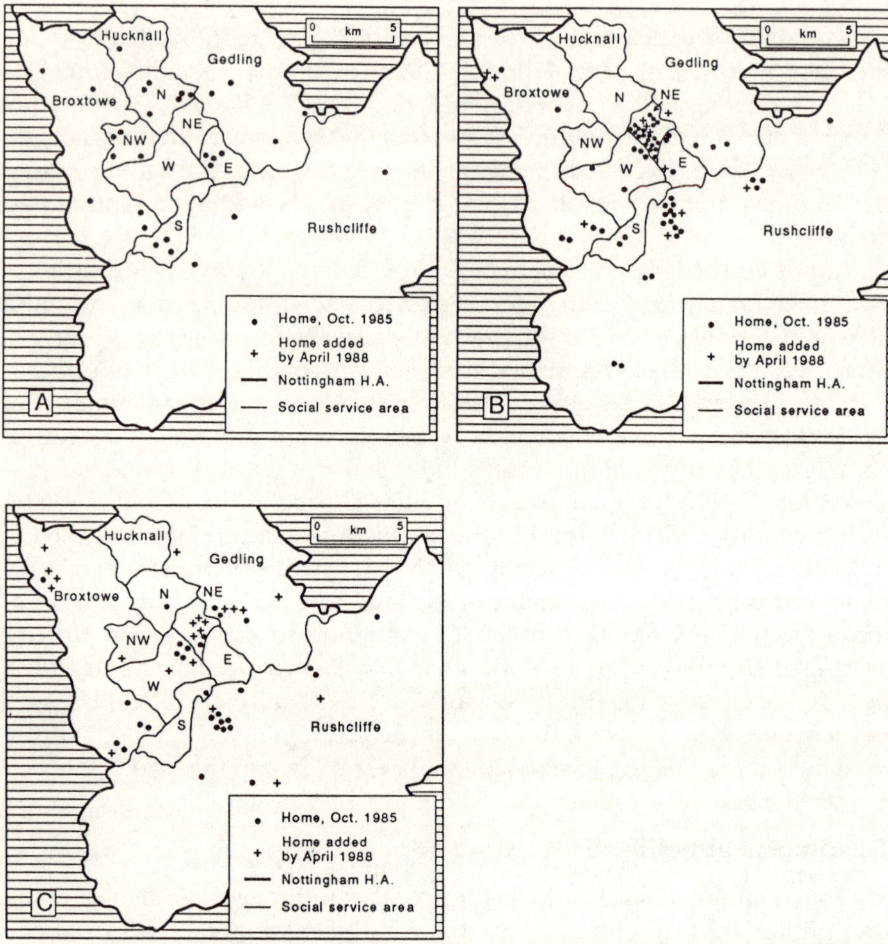

Source: Nottingham County Council 1985; Nottingham Health Authority 1985

*Figure 7.1: Distribution of homes for the elderly in Nottingham Health Authority (England): A) Part III (Local Authority) homes; B) Private rest homes; C) Private nursing homes; October 1985–April 1988 **

From the map and table it becomes apparent that heavily populated areas of Nottingham City, such as Mapperley, Mapperley Park and Sherwood (all within Nottingham NE social service area) and New Basford, Radford, Lenton, Dunkirk and Wollaton (all within Nottingham W social service area) appear to have had no local Part III provision at all. Conversely, Nottingham N (including areas such as Bulwell and Bestwood) and Nottingham S (mainly Clifton) areas had actual provision levels that were above 30 places per 1000 elderly people, i.e. over twice the average for the HA.

Table 7.1: Distribution of elderly population and places in Social Service areas; Nottingham Health Authority, England (October 1985)

		Nottingham						*Nottingham*			
	Rushcliffe	*Broxtowe*	*Gedling*	*Hucknall*	*N*	*NW*	*NE*	*W*	*E*	*S*	*HA (total)*
Population, 65+	12,939	14,120	13,395	3257	8410	7008	6810	8390	6647	4028	85,274
Part III Homes											
Homes	3	4	4	1	6	4	0	0	4	3	29
Places	165	187	181	50	300	156	0	0	194	134	1,367
Places/1000	12.75	13.24	13.51	15.35	35.67	22.26	0	0	29.12	33.26	16.03
Private rest homes											
Homes	19	6	3	0	0	0	22	6	3	3	62
Places	257	88	42	0	0	0	324	159	74	63	1,007
Places/1000	19.86	6.23	3.14	0	0	0	47.58	18.95	11.13	15.64	11.81
Private nursing homes											
Homes	12	4	3	0	0	0	2	4	0	1	26
Places	314	98	71	0	0	0	34	155	0	14	686
Places/1000	24.27	6.98	5.30	0	0	0	4.99	18.47	0	3.48	8.04
Total residential											
Accommodation											
Homes	34	14	10	1	6	4	24	10	7	7	117
Places	736	373	294	50	300	156	358	314	268	211	3,060
Places/1000	56.88	26.41	21.95	15.35	35.67	22.26	52.56	37.43	40.32	52.38	35.88
(% Part III)	22	50	62	100	100	100	0	0	72	64	45

Source: Notts County Council (1981), Notts County Council (1985), Nottingham Health Authority (1985), OPCS (1983)

In addition to this problem of discrepant availability of Part III places, a further difficulty was that old people may actually have been placed within the same social service area but much further from their old homes and neighbourhoods than if they were placed across a social service boundary much nearer to their original homes. This created obvious problems with regard to visits by friends and relatives and access by old people to their home neighbourhoods. Moreover, in the few years before 1985 the number of Part III places available locally had increased very slightly as a result of three new homes opening, but government spending restrictions in place by 1985 rendered future Part III openings as extremely unlikely. Indeed by 1985 government policy clearly favoured the private sector and attendant growth in numbers of private rest and nursing homes.

Data kindly provided by the Nottinghamshire Social Services Department (1985) have permitted a similar map to be constructed summarising the distribution of the 62 private rest homes located within the Nottingham HA in October 1985 (see Figure 7.1B). These data include only those homes with more than four residents and exclude rest homes catering for non-elderly residents. It is evident that the geographical distribution of the private rest homes was completely different from that of Part III local authority homes. Broadly, two main concentrations occurred: in the Nottingham NE social service area, principally in the Mapperley Park and Sherwood areas (22 homes); and in the Rushcliffe social service area, where there are 19 homes of which 11 are found in West Bridgford. The conclusion must be that these two concentrations reflected the type of housing stock available in the two areas; large detached houses that might otherwise have been divided into flat units are commonplace in both areas and were the favoured accommodation for private rest homes.

Conversely, Nottingham N, Nottingham NW and Hucknall had no private rest homes at all, whilst the remaining five social service areas had numbers varying between two and six. It is clear, therefore, that the spatial distribution of private rest homes in October 1985 was very uneven; Table 7.1 summarises these inequalities. One alarming feature was that suitable private rest homes may not have been available locally for elderly residents, thus necessitating their movement to West Bridgford or Sherwood. Once again, the issue of visiting by relatives and friends was seen to be a potential problem. Moreover, poorer areas such as Hucknall and Bilborough (in Nottingham NW area) were totally devoid of private rest homes.

The changing numbers of private rest home places within the Nottingham HA catchment area are summarised in Figure 7.2. Here they are divided into voluntary rest-home places (such as Methodist homes for the aged), for which figures had remained fairly stable at about 300 places over the five years up to October 1985, and profit-making private rest homes, for which 1980–85 saw a change from 170 to around 730 places, an increase of about 430% in five years.

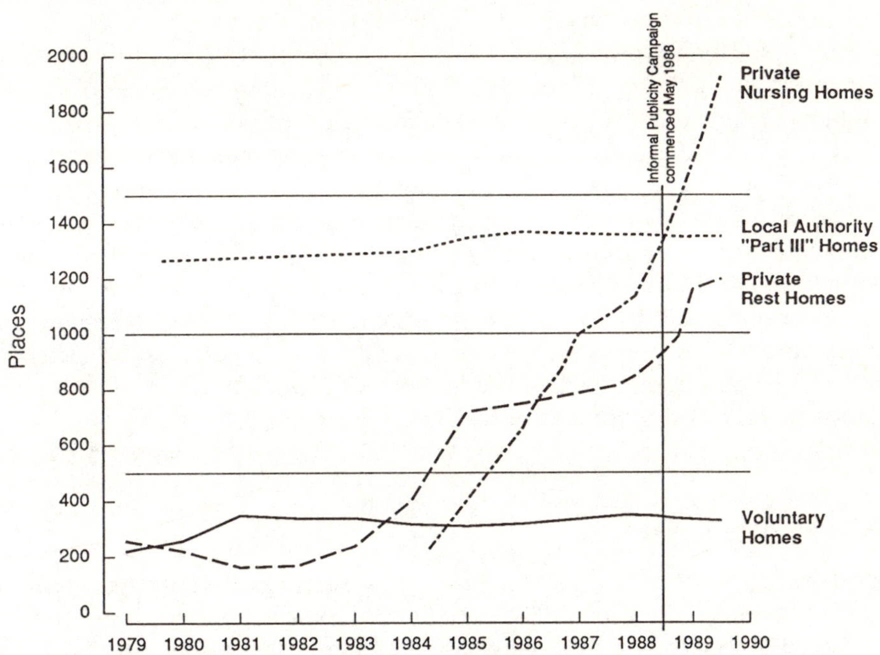

Source: Nottinghamshire County Council 1985; Nottingham Health Authority 1989)

*Figure 7.2: Changing trends in residential care for the elderly in Nottingham Health Authority (England) 1979–1989 **

The private nursing home sector also experienced a major explosion in the four years before October 1985. Using data kindly provided by the Nottingham HA (1985), the geographical distribution of, and provision levels for, these homes were assessed. However, the rapidly expanding private nursing home sector in Nottingham by 1985 made an entirely accurate summary difficult. Figure 7.1C summarises the spatial distribution of the 26 nursing homes within the Nottingham HA which were accepting elderly residents in October 1985, whilst Table 7.1 provides a summary of provision levels for the local elderly population.

Once again, certain spatial concentrations were obvious: West Bridgford's housing stock, as in the case of rest homes, was clearly responsible for the seven homes concentrated in that area. Indeed, the Rushcliffe social service area generally boasted a level of nursing home places that was three times the average for the entire HA. The second concentration occurred in the Forest Fields and Sherwood Rise areas, at the extreme eastern end of the large Nottingham W social service area. This is adjacent to Mapperley Park, where so many private rest homes are concentrated. Again one must suggest that the local housing stock was the major factor associated with this concentration; the level of nursing home places within Nottingham W was thus over twice the average for the health authority in October 1985.

Four of the ten areas had no private nursing homes at all, including poorer areas such as Hucknall, Bilborough (in Nottingham N) and Sneinton (Nottingham E). One must reiterate that spatial concentration of homes in a few areas may necessitate movement of elderly patients over considerable distances and can create attendant problems for visiting friends and relatives.

The numbers of private nursing homes in the Nottingham HA was increasing almost monthly during the mid-1980s. This growth is summarised in Figure 7.2; in April 1984 there were 260 places, by October 1985 there were 686, and by June 1986 it had reached 1009. This represented a nearly fourfold increase in a little over two years. In addition, at October 1985 a further 11 homes with 343 beds were scheduled for completion by the following June and a number of further planning applications were under consideration.

The Situation in 1985

The rapid growth of the private residential sector nationally had excited much interest by the mid-1980s. A review of national and regional trends produced at that time by Larder *et al* (1985) noted that public provision by local authority was highest in the north and lowest in the south, with the midlands in the middle of the range. Conversely, voluntary and especially private provisions were highest in the south and lowest in the north. This north-south divide was attributed to the greater wealth of the southern part of Britain and, in addition, to the greater concentration of elderly people in the coastal areas of the south. Another noted feature was the political orientation of local councils in the different parts of the country, with the associated north-south variations. However, since Labour councils predominate in poorer areas and Conservative councils in richer ones, this was hardly surprising.

Nationally, Larder *et al* maintained that the social security system, which offered access to private nursing and residential care, might provide enough incentives for the private sector to 'move into the presently under-provided (and perhaps less wealthy) parts of the country', though they remained rather doubtful about the possibility, given that many parts of Britain had a low level of wealth. They noted with concern that merely allowing market forces to influence the development of a mixed public/private residential system would not in itself actually lead to a more equal distribution of provision. There were two possible policy implications to be drawn from this: first, that planning regulations could be tightened up to control the private sector more; conversely, the second was that given difficulties of defining provision norms, equity could best be achieved by distributing more equally the ability to choose between types of homes rather than aiming at an equal distribution of provision.

Of course the weakness of the latter argument has already been made clear above in the Nottingham context: merely giving people the ability to move into a residential home somewhere does not necessarily 'democratise' access for relatives and friends, given that the residential unit may be some distance from the home neighbourhood. This may equally be the case in both private and statutory homes, but planning regulation and more equal geographical distribution of the former relative to the elderly population throughout the community would ease the problem.

The need for planning was discussed in a local context by Phillips and Vincent (1986) and Phillips *et al* (1987) in their detailed study of private residential accommodation in Devon. Whilst noting that the availability of buildings suitable for conversion to private old people's homes was more common in certain areas, they concluded that 'a largely undirected and potentially unstable' private sector did not provide a sound basis for meeting the needs of the nation's elderly population. Whilst suggesting that a planning component sounded a plausible alternative, British planning regulations were not well suited to regulating the growth of the industry; instead they are more concerned with land-use criteria, final applications for building conversions, technical standards of access, fire regulations and parking provision, and are not really concerned with the demographic composition of a neighbourhood, or the actual 'needs' of the elderly population therein (Ross 1985).

Assessing and Meeting Needs

This leads to the issue of assessing 'need' in the context of the elderly. Here Blake (1968) suggested that vaguely-worded legislation does not actually do very much to reduce variations between different areas, since interpretation of 'need' varies greatly between different local authorities in fields such as residential homes. Thus, she argued, local policy decisions regarding provision levels of residential accommodation should ultimately be regarded as political. Yet even within the Nottingham HA in the mid-1980s significant local variations had already been noted in the three types of residential home assessed. When the provision levels are combined to provide an overall picture of the then residential accommodation for the elderly (see Table 7.1) then that spatial variation persisted. Given an average overall level of around 36 places per 1000 elderly people for the HA, and remembering that this average level was likely to rise abruptly as more private homes were built in the richer areas, the two relatively poor areas of Hucknall and Gedling (including Arnold and Carlton) had the lowest provision levels relative to their elderly populations. Moreover, Hucknall managed only one home in total, and that was a Part III one, whilst two-thirds of Gedling's places were also Part III type. Two other areas – Broxtowe and Nottingham NW – fell below the HA average, with a high proportion of their places made by the statutory sector.

By contrast, richer areas such as Rushcliffe (including West Bridgford) and Nottingham NE (including Mapperley Park) had much higher than average place allocations and very low (22 % and zero respectively) statutory place contributions. In the cases of Nottingham N, E and S social service areas, however, provision levels at or above the average were achieved, with a majority of the places offered being statutory. Whilst these areas clearly did not have a housing stock that favoured private sector development, it was encouraging that provision levels had remained so high. However, at this time it was thought that these levels would certainly fall back speedily as the private sector expanded elsewhere and increased the average provision level. Furthermore, the demographic ageing effect in the three areas would also, over time, act to lower the respective provision levels still further.

Local Developments in the Late 1980s

The further development of residential accommodation for the elderly within the Nottingham HA was monitored continuously throughout the period October 1985 – June 1989. By April 1988 (i.e. 30 months after the initial survey) there were an extra 32 private homes and 937 places (see Tables 7.2 and 7.3); however the same inequality between the more affluent areas (i.e. Rushcliffe and Nottingham NE) and the poorer areas remained. Indeed these two concentrations appear to have been exaggerated further in this 30 month period, whilst there were areas further north with little or no provision at either date (Figure 7.1 illustrates the local distribution of rest and nursing homes present by October 1985 and those added by April 1988). Since October 1985 there have been no further developments at all – either openings or closures – in the local Part III sector.

By May 1988 the HA had established a working party to observe the local private sector in some detail. In the absence of any statutory controls over the opening of new private homes on grounds of local need, it was decided to attempt a publicity campaign to inform potential and existing home owners about the distribution of these existing homes. It was suggested that this might encourage new developments in previously ignored areas, whilst appealing to the business instincts of these developers to take advantage of previously untapped 'markets'. Initially a series of seminars was organised to which local owners were invited; information sheets were made available at this and subsequent meetings.

In the 12 months following the commencement of this campaign (ie June 1988 – June 1989) a total of 12 rest and 11 nursing homes opened within the HA (see Tables 7.4 and 7.5). Some developments occurred in peripheral areas (e.g. Hucknall) but many were concentrated in the same old areas. In this 12 month period about 600 new places appeared. And by June 1989 overall provision was nearly 5000 places in Part III, rest and nursing homes for a total of about 85,000 elderly people (about 5.7 %); this figure excludes elderly

Table 7.2: Distribution of elderly population and places in Social Service areas; Nottingham Health Authority, England (April 1988)

			Nottingham					Nottingham			
	Rushcliffe	*Broxtowe*	*Gedling*	*Hucknall*	*N*	*NW*	*NE*	*W*	*E*	*S*	*HA (total)*
Population, 65+	12,939	14,120	13,395	3257	8410	7008	6810	8390	6647	4028	85,274
Part III Homes											
Homes	3	4	4	1	6	4	0	0	4	3	29
Places	165	187	181	50	300	156	0	0	194	134	1,367
Places/1000	12.75	13.24	13.51	15.35	35.67	22.26	0	0	29.12	33.26	16.03
Private rest homes											
Homes	22	9	4	0	0	0	24	6	4	3	72
Places	324	167	59	0	0	0	363	177	118	64	1,271
Places/1000	25.04	11.63	4.40	0	0	0	53.30	21.09	17.75	15.88	14.90
Private nursing homes											
Homes	15	9	8	0	1	1	7	6	0	1	48
Places	508	202	201	0	18	24	148	243	0	14	1,358
Places/1000	39.26	14.31	15.00	0	2.14	3.42	21.73	28.96	0	3.48	15.93
Total accommodation											
Homes	40	22	16	1	7	5	31	12	8	7	149
Places	997	556	441	50	318	180	511	420	312	212	3,997
Places/1000	77.05	39.38	32.92	15.35	37.81	25.68	75.04	50.05	46.94	52.63	46.87
(% Part III)	17	34	41	100	94	87	0	0	62	63	34

Source: Notts County Council (1988), Nottingham Health Authority (1988), OPCS (1983)

Table 7.3. Changes in the provision of accommodation for the elderly; Nottingham Health Authority, England (October 1985 – April 1988)

		Nottingham						*Nottingham*			
	Rushcliffe	*Broxtowe*	*Gedling*	*Hucknall*	*N*	*NW*	*NE*	*W*	*E*	*S*	*HA (total)*
Part III Homes											
Homes	0	0	0	0	0	0	0	0	0	0	0
Places	0	0	0	0	0	0	0	0	0	0	0
Places/1000	0	0	0	0	0	0	0	0	0	0	0
Private rest homes											
Homes	+3	+3	+1	0	0	0	+2	0	+1	0	+10
Places	+67	+79	+17	0	0	0	+39	+18	+44	+1	+265
Places/1000	+5.18	+5.40	+1.26	0	0	0	+5.72	+2.14	+6.62	+0.26	+3.09
Private nursing homes											
Homes	+3	+5	+5	0	+1	+1	+5	+2	0	0	+22
Places	+194	+104	+130	0	+18	+24	+114	+88	0	0	+672
Places/1000	14.99	7.33	9.70	0	+2.14	+3.42	+16.74	+10.49	0	0	+7.89
Total residential Accommodation											
Homes	+6	+8	+6	0	+1	+1	+7	+2	+1	0	+32
Places	+261	+183	+147	0	+18	+24	+153	+106	+44	+1	+937
Places/1000	+20.17	+12.97	+10.97	0	+2.14	+3.42	+22.48	+12.64	+6.62	+0.25	+10.99
(% Part III)	-5	-16	-21	0	-6	-13	0	0	-10	-1	-11

Source: Notts County Council (1988), Nottingham Health Authority (1988), OPCS (1983)

Table 7.4. Distribution of elderly population and places in Social Service areas; Nottingham Health Authority, England (June 1989)

		Nottingham						*Nottingham*			
	Rushcliffe	*Broxtowe*	*Gedling*	*Hucknall*	*N*	*NW*	*NE*	*W*	*E*	*S*	*HA (total)*
Population, 65+	12,939	14,120	13,395	3257	8410	7008	6810	8390	6647	4028	85,274
Part III Homes											
Homes	3	4	4	1	6	4	0	0	4	3	29
Places	165	187	181	50	300	156	0	0	194	134	1,367
Places/1000	12.75	13.24	13.51	15.35	35.67	22.26	0	0	29.12	33.26	6.03
Private rest homes											
Homes	24	14	4	2	0	0	31	9	4	3	91
Places	374	274	59	19	0	0	425	213	118	64	1,546
Places/1000	28.90	19.41	4.40	5.83	0	0	62.41	25.39	17.75	15.88	18.13
Private nursing homes											
Homes	16	14	16	1	3	1	8	6	0	1	66
Places	601	357	376	35	98	24	184	243	0	14	1,932
Places/1000	46.45	25.28	28.07	10.75	11.65	3.42	27.02	28.96	0	3.48	22.66
Total accommodation											
Homes	43	32	24	4	9	5	39	15	8	7	186
Places	1,140	818	616	104	398	180	609	456	312	212	4,845
Places/1000	88.11	57.93	45.99	31.93	47.32	25.68	89.43	54.35	46.94	52.63	56.82
(% Part III)	15	23	29	48	75	87	0	0	62	63	28

Source: *Notts County Council (1988), Nottingham Health Authority (1988), OPCS (1983)*

Table 7.5. Changing distribution of accommodation for the elderly; Nottingham Health Authority, England (June 1988 – June 1989)

			Nottingham				*Nottingham*				
	Rushcliffe	*Broxtowe*	*Gedling*	*Hucknall*	*N*	*NW*	*NE*	*W*	*E*	*S*	*HA (total)*
Part III Homes											
Homes	0	0	0	0	0	0	0	0	0	0	0
Places	0	0	0	0	0	0	0	0	0	0	0
Private rest homes											
Homes	+2	+2	0	+1	0	0	+5	+2	0	0	+12
Places	+50	+47	0	+8	0	0	+48	+30	0	0	+183
Private nursing homes											
Homes	0	+4	+3	+1	+2	0	+1	0	0	0	+11
Places	+72	+127	+63	+35	+80	0	+36	0	0	0	+413
Total new accommodation											
Homes	+2	+6	+3	+2	+2	0	+6	+2	0	0	+23
Places	+122	+174	+63	+43	+80	0	+84	+30	0	0	+596

Source: Notts County Council (1988, 1989); Nottingham Health Authority (1988, 1989); OPCS (1983)

people in hospitals. However changes in this 12 month period appear to have produced very little harmonisation in provision levels between different areas (see Figure 7.3); put another way, the informal publicity campaign appears not to have been a major success, though some modest developments in some needy areas had started by mid-1989.

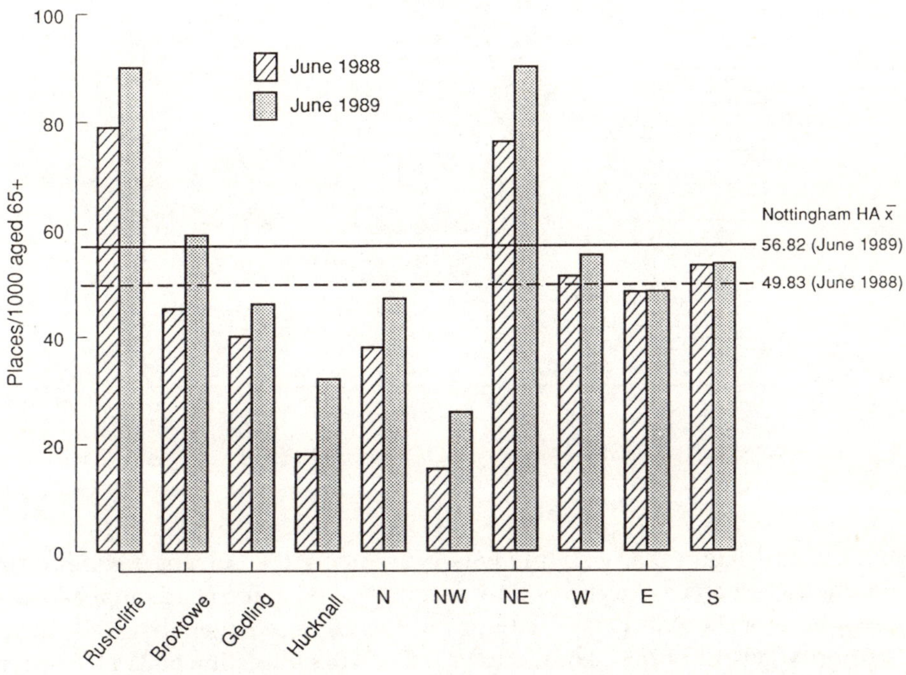

Figure 7.3: Total accomodation provision (Part III, rest and nursing homes) by Social Service Area, 1988–1989

Conclusions

The mapping of residential developments for elderly people around Nottingham has revealed a very uneven geographical distribution of private developments relative to actual local elderly populations; this trend has actually widened between richer and poorer areas since 1985, with homes being established primarily in two more affluent parts of the city with many inner city and peripheral areas receiving scant provision. Specific conclusions are made in Figure 7.4 regarding the required direction of future developments locally, made on the basis of existing homes and numbers of elderly people locally.

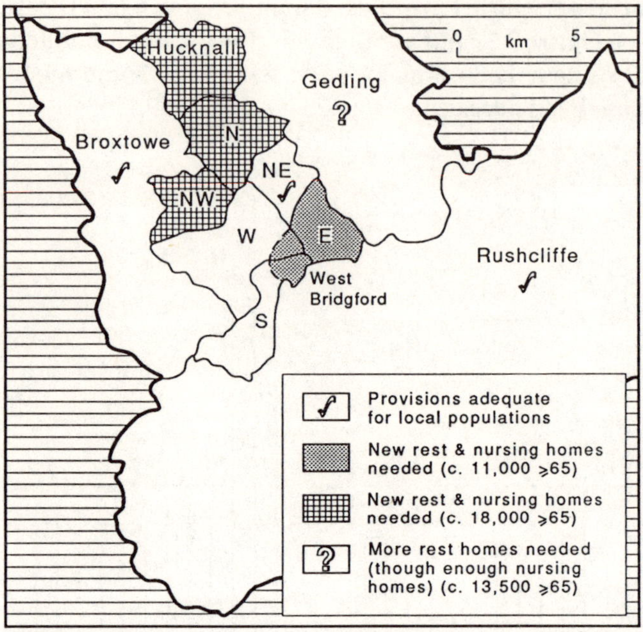

Figure 7.4: Suggested optimal development of residual accomodation in Nottingham (England)

But can one suggest any simple way of reducing the current inequalities? Before the expansion of the private sector, provision for residential accommodation for the elderly population was, to a large extent, managed by local authority Part III homes. For many years a DHSS guideline of 25 places per 1000 elderly (65+ years) was used, though there was no statutory obligation for local authorities to conform to this standard. In reality few did; for example in Nottingham provision of Part III places stood at abut 15 per 1000 elderly people for many years. Were an updated system of recommended provision levels for both private and statutory homes introduced, it would be impossible for local social services and health authorities to reinforce it without the right to veto possible private developments in favour of others in more appropriate areas. No such veto power exists. It is hardly current government policy to give statutory powers to local social services or health authorities to control private sector developments; thus statutory guidelines are very unlikely in the foreseeable political climate.

A more sophisticated measure than the older DHSS guideline would be desirable, perhaps based upon numbers of very elderly people (say aged 75+ years) by census ward or similar small geographical unit, with additional inputs of local census data measuring disability and disadvantage. This could be worked into a simple though effective scale of need and then applied by a local licensing body, consisting for example of officers from both health authority and social services acting together. And especially if this measure was statutory and not voluntary. Thus potential developers would be allowed to open new homes only when a genuine local need existed and not just when it is convenient for the developer.

In the meanwhile one is left to monitor private developments locally and to encourage growth in certain areas of need. Following upon the series of seminars organised by the Nottingham HA, licensing officers in both the HA and Notts. County Council are now showing maps of distribution of existing homes to potential developers and pointing out areas of low provision by suggesting that these are an important and as yet untapped local market.

However, responses from the private sector to these informal approaches have, as noted above, been very muted, and the feeling encouraged that approaching owners of existing homes through a series of seminars is not the most efficient way of encouraging the better siting of future homes. Conversely, the expansion of corporate involvement in the private sector – involving ownership of multiple homes by large companies – is now growing within the private system, initially in the south of England, but more recently in the Midlands, and the possibility exists that a more professional business approach would want to take advantage of the now well demonstrated inequalities and exploit specific local markets (Laing and Buisson 1988).

Ultimately, one must question just how long the private sector will continue to expand, bearing in mind the recent demographic ageing effects – which although substantial will certainly not be infinite – and the future likelihood or otherwise of continued and significant government (i.e. DSS) funding of the private sector. In parts of southern England the rate of growth of this private sector is now slowing, though currently there is little sign of this in the East Midlands: one wonders just how soon levelling-out will begin.

If, as seems likely, some ceiling is reached locally within the next couple of years – and in September 1989 there were 150 unoccupied nursing home places in Nottingham to encourage this levelling out – then one must worry about the likely long-term inequalities existing within overall provision for elderly people. If the market reaches a point of stagnation, then existing inequalities may become permanent, whilst if, or when, government funding became tighter, then one could foresee bankruptcy, or at least partial withdrawal from the private residential sector as profitability declined, with serious consequences for the vulnerable elderly people unfortunate enough to be affected directly.

In the long term, therefore, one must question just how stable the local private residential market is, especially so when so many homes are concentrated in so few places and are therefore chasing a geographically concentrated and limited potential clientele. If or when the changed conditions described above occur then we could foresee serious local problems arising, with an attendant effect of increasing waiting lists for council-run Part III places, the slowing of discharge rates from hospital geriatric beds and the associated 'bed blocking' in hospitals so common just a few years ago.

Demographic ageing effects over the last few years – in association with government policies to encourage the business community – have nurtured a rapid growth of private developments both nationally and locally. In the long term, however, one must suggest a move towards a more controlled and co-ordinated environment consisting of a mix of private and statutory accommodation. By the turn of the century the proportion of very elderly people in our population will be much higher; the need will exist, therefore, for a permanent and stable residential accommodation sector that is regulated properly and inspected thoroughly.

To ignore current inequalities and potential problems locally is really to ignore likely future problems; these will eventually have to be addressed and a move made towards realistic and statutory planning mechanisms designed centrally but implemented locally. Bearing in mind that the Nottingham HA has been the subject of an ongoing study of the private sector, and considering that this local area is in many ways typical of much of the country, then continued work in Nottingham may point the way for the future.

Acknowledgments

The author is grateful to Mrs D.M. Currie, Nurse Advisor, Nottingham HA, and Dr N. Nice, Service Planning Manager, Nottingham HA, for data relating to private nursing homes and hospitals. The Social Services Department at Nottinghamshire County Council provided data on private rest homes and Part III places. Demographic data were provided partly by the Planning Department, also at Nottinghamshire County Council. The author is especially grateful to Professor T. Arie and Dr K. Morgan (both, Department of Health Care of the Elderly, Nottingham University) and to Mr K. Grant (Division of Geography, Thames Valley University) for their encouragement in the preparation of this chapter. The manuscript was kindly typed by Ms Jenny Johns and the diagrams kindly prepared by Mr John Williamson.

References

Carson, D. (1985) Registering homes: another fine mess? *Journal of Social Welfare Law* 7, 67–84.

Challis, L. (1982) *Private and voluntary residential provision for the elderly: report of an exploratory study of residential and nursing homes in the City of Bath.* Centre for the Analysis of Social Policy: University of Bath.

DHSS (1981) *Care in the Community: a consultative document on moving resources for care in England.* London: HMSO.

Laing and Buisson (1988) *Care of Elderly People.* London: Laing and Buisson Publications Ltd.

Larder, D. et al (1986) *Institutional care for the elderly: the geographical distribution of the public/private mix in England.* Centre for the Analysis of Social Policy: University of Bath.

Mears, K. and Smith, R. (1985) *The Development of Welfare Services for Elderly People.* London: Croom Helm.

Nottingham Health Authority (1985) Unpublished quarterly report of registered nursing homes.

Nottinghamshire County Council (1982) *Population Report 1981.* Nottingham: Director of Planning and Transportation.

Nottinghamshire County Council (1985) *Registered residential homes within Nottinghamshire* Nottingham.

OPCS (1976) *Population projection 1974–2014.* London: HMSO.

OPCS (1983) *Census 1981 – County Report: Nottinghamshire Part I.* London: HMSO.

Phillips, D. R. and Vincent, J. A. (1986) Private residential accommodation for the elderly: geographical aspects of developments in Devon, *Transaction Institute of British Geographers N.S.* 11, 155–173.

Phillips, D. R. et al (1987) Spatial concentration of residential homes for the elderly: planning responses and dilemmas. *Transactions Institute of British Geographers N.S.* 12, 73–83

Ross, R. B. (1985) Regulation of residential homes for the elderly in England and Wales. *Journal of Social Welfare Law* 7, 85–95

CHAPTER 8

Health Economists and Health Care Provision for the Elderly

Implicit Assumptions and Unstated Conclusions

Ian R. Jones and Paul F.D. Higgs

The impact of Health Economics is now all apparent. Steadily over the past decade the focus of policy debate in the British health and social services has shifted from the idea of universalism to the search for cost-efficiency and 'value-for-money'. Hospital and community services have been reformed in the image of the classical economic 'firm' and now talk openly of 'business plans'. This transformation has been achieved partly by means of the Griffiths management report of 1983 which involved the creation of general management and devolved budget holding; but overwhelmingly by the White Paper 'Working for Patients' (now the NHS Act of 1990) which conceived of a restructured health care system as a bounded form of the classical economic market.

In Britain this is mirrored in local government where, throughout the 1980s, social services departments were subject to the financial austerity of government-imposed limitations on their budgets ('rate-capping'). Now they are to be given new roles under the community care legislation; roles which will see them acting as agent purchasers of care for client groups and which will allow private contractors full opportunity to 'bid' for the provision of services on the basis of price and quality. Other public sector organisations will also be able to offer their services for a price and vice versa, creating a much more complex interface between the NHS and local government.

This organisational and political transformation has also led to the increased importance of individual health economists. Their role in planning, assessing and evaluating health care has become accepted in many health authorities; under competition this role will become even more acute with each unit needing to develop a market strategy.

If health economics is the future of health care in Britain then the well known demographic changes in the age structure of the population will be the background of many of the decisions influenced by health economists.

It is therefore important that those involved in social gerontology have an awareness of how old age is viewed in health economics and how elderly people can be discriminated against by the use of these ideas in health care decision making. It is also important that health economists and others are alerted to the implicit assumptions and unstated conclusions of mainstream health economic theory.

This chapter will outline the various methods used by health economists to evaluate health care options. It will show how they all share a common theoretical tradition and how this perspective can have a negative impact on the health care received by older people. It will conclude with a call for the construction of an alternative set of values as a basis for the rational delivery of health care.

The Perspective of Health Economics

It is commonplace to point out that economics is not a value-free discipline. Indeed, the various schools of thought that make up the discipline disagree on a whole host of key ideas. The development, transformation into orthodoxy and counter-revolution against (and now resurrection of) Keynesian macroeconomic [1] thought that has occurred over the past 30 years is a clear example that even the workings of the market are not universally agreed upon by economists. Within health economics there is a similar difference of opinion towards the nature of health care as an economic system. This implies that no one model of economic rationality is definitive or has all the answers.

The motivation behind the discipline of health economics lies in wanting to develop 'rational' tools for the planning and evaluation of health care. Behind this lies the desire to minimise decision-making being made on the basis of individual value judgements or as a continuation of time honoured practice. What is important to health economics is that the full consequences of allocative and operational decisions are acknowledged and that the basis of decision-making is 'explicit'.

> ...the economic approach to rationing is explicit: it makes what is at present inconsistent, incoherent and implicit, open to democratic review. (Maynard 1990, p.188)

However, within the ideas and articulations of mainstream health economics theory this 'openness' is often forgotten or excluded. Simple neo-classical rationality is imputed in all decision making. Concepts such as need are quantified from the perspective of the providers (the health authority / firm) and analytic tools such as value are borrowed from the disciplines of actuarial science and accountancy.

Economic rationality based on classical economic theories is not intrinsically wrong, but it is limited in its horizons. It may adequately describe the resource implications of decisions but cannot take into consideration the wider role of health care, or if it does it often finds itself in contradiction with this wider role. Acceptance that health economics is not value free or neutral also implies that some of the methods used can have a negative impact on certain groups in the population.

This is especially important if these methods of economic evaluation contain hidden value judgements about the form of care that should or should not be made available to certain groups at a given cost. Avorn points out that many of the methods employed by health economists

> ...embody a set of hidden value assumptions that virtually guarantee an anti-geriatric bias to this purportedly objective data. (Avorn 1984, p.1295)

He goes on to argue that the attraction of health economics is that it promises to solve difficult allocative decisions by means of 'a standardised set of algorithms' as well as fitting in with 'the corporatisation of health care'. This is the case because in borrowing neo-classical ideas and models from the philosophy of utilitarianism[2], much of health economics simultaneously brings into it's work the assumptions of productive worth on which these models are based.

It therefore introduces its own set of implicit value judgements. It is not the intention of most health economists to act in this way, for most recognise that implicit value judgements can lead to bad decisions. But unfortunately, because the models they use are based upon these neo-classical definitions of economic worth, implicit value judgements are built into the very procedures of rational decision making. This tendency is accentuated when professionals unversed in economic theory utilise the tools given to them by health economics in an unknowing way.

The Principle Idea: Opportunity Cost

Economically rational decisions are those that maximise the benefits gained from the use of resources. If resources are finite then competing claims on those resources have to be weighed up and appropriate action taken. Within the classical firm these decisions are taken in terms of which course of action offers the best return on investment. Within the field of health care these same decisions are also made; albeit there may be differences between whether it is cost or human benefit that is the objective.

What is really being described is the concept of opportunity cost, which must have a major role in health care decision making if health care is to become rational. The importance of such an idea cannot be overstated as many clinicians, as well as other professionals, exhibit (as far as health economists are concerned) unknowingly wasteful behaviour through their lack of knowledge of the consequences of their decisions. However, opportunity costs – i.e. benefits foregone from adopting one course of action instead of another – are often only seen in the context of calls on health service revenues. Indeed, the attempt to encourage care by informal carers is one example where an understanding of the opportunity cost of withdrawal from the labour market by an individual carer is acknowledged but is not quantified.

The above ideas illustrate the dilemmas that can be produced by an uncritical use of health economic theory. In the rush to discipline clinicians and managers alike with economic rationality, the dangers of using what is at best a blunt tool are often forgotten, with particular implications for the more vulnerable sections of society.

In the USA there is much discussion of an intergenerational crisis (Callahan 1987, Churchill 1986) where the elderly, as high users of resources, are seen as having fundamentally opposed interests to the rest of society. Similar arguments have been advanced in this country most notably in the collection *Workers Versus Pensioners* (Johnson, Conrad and Thomson 1989). Although these are extreme arguments they fit in with other currents in the health economics literature in their emphasis on the non-productivity of the elderly and their role as economic burden.

What we intend to do in the next section is to show how a number of different methods of economic evaluation can lead to discrimination against elderly people.

Cost Benefit Analysis

Cost Benefit Analysis (CBA) is the economic tool that is most contentious within the field of health care. It equates health care with any other commodity, seeing it purely in terms of costed inputs and outputs. In other words, it quantifies both the costs of a health care intervention and the outcomes of that intervention in monetary terms. The analysis is based on the concept of efficiency which is defined by McGuire *et al* (1988) as: 'A state where the costs of producing a given output are minimised and the utility of individual's preferences are maximised' (McGuire, Henderson and Mooney 1988, p.287).

It is here that the contradiction between economics and health care is most apparent. Whilst it is obviously in everybody's interest to organise health care as rationally as possible, CBA exists in order to create a surrogate market environment for health services. It does so because of its belief that market-type decision making is the only way to make truly rational decisions. In this the economic tool is very close to its neo-classical theoretical roots. It perceives the operation of economics as inevitably leading to the satisfaction of need at the optimal cost. This is because the market system operates so that all markets tend towards equilibrium, maximising inputs and outputs.

Neo-classical economic theory argues that the market mechanism can achieve a balance of efficiency between costs and needs. This is known as Pareto efficiency (see McGuire *et al* 1988), where a stated amount of resources creates an optimum position of efficiency at a point where it is impossible to make one individual better off without making another individual worse off. In this way both 'supplier' and 'buyer' benefit; with the supplier providing health care at the most rational level and the buyers having their needs met.

In the real world, however, and particularly with respect to health care, markets are imperfect and do not achieve a balance. CBA can therefore be described as a response to such imperfections in that it tries to identify those projects that satisfy the criteria of what McGuire *et al* call 'potential pareto improvement'. To do this the analysis tries to identify all the costs and benefits associated with a project so that its efficiency can be compared with that of other projects. The principle being that inefficient projects are discarded and efficient projects are accepted. Such an analysis has immense potential for assisting in decision making and informing comprehensive plans for allocating resources on a systematic basis. However, problems arise when one looks at the concept of efficiency and how this is defined by economists.

Efficiency

Social efficiency exists when the total value of outputs produced is maximised and it is impossible to make one person better off without making another worse off. It is this approach that underpins the use of CBA techniques. In many studies currently undertaken the criteria are adapted so that only aggregate social efficiency is adopted.

Under a project that increases social efficiency, so defined, it is possible for some individuals to be made worse off; i.e. as long as the total value of outputs produced is increased it does not matter what happens to individuals within the equation. The point is encapsulated by Williams (1985) when he argues:

> The objective of economic appraisal is to ensure that as much benefit as possible is obtained from the resources devoted to health care. (Williams 1985, p.326)

Such an analysis is simplistic; indeed, it is not difficult to take it to its logical extreme and conceive of a socially efficient situation where the elderly receive little resource because the benefit gained from directing resources to them is less than that gained from directing it to other younger groups (this point is made by Evans 1990). As a counterpoint to this happening, McGuire *et al* (1988) argue that equity and distribution must also be included in economic appraisal if it is to produce a comprehensive social welfare function. Therefore it is important that the needs of all of the population (especially the elderly) have to be taken into consideration irrespective of whether these are 'efficient' in CBA terms or not.

CBA is flawed because it ignores these distributional issues of equity, fairness and allocative justice. Under the objective set by Williams (1985) its results will merely reflect the unfairness and inefficiencies that already exist in society.

Cost Effectiveness Analysis

Cost Effectiveness Analysis (CEA) differs from CBA in that it attempts to give managers different options of achieving the same end. It exists on its own rather than as an applied version of a larger macroeconomic theory. CEA evaluates projects in terms of technical efficiency whereby projects are accepted if they maximise benefits at a given cost or alternatively minimise the cost of achieving a particular outcome. Cost Utility Analysis (CUA) is a variant of CEA which compares the incremental cost of a programme with the resulting incremental health improvement measured in Quality Adjusted Life Years (QALYS), which are fully discussed below.

CEA and CUA do not have the same theoretical problems as CBA but as Brooks (1985) points out they do have similar technical problems including how to value intangibles such as well-being. These problems increase if the patient group being studied has a multiplicity of clinical problems. This is because one side of the equation must be kept constant; either this must be the objectives of the service (which implies no limit on the resources available to achieve it) or the resources available (which implies fixing the needs at a certain level). Nowhere is this more true than when the elderly are under scrutiny. Their needs are often manifold and consequently there is a tendency to package their needs to existing staffing or resource levels. The impact of CEA for services for the elderly is to see to what extent needs can be met with prospectively limited budgets. In addition, the analysis has a tendency to define what needs are rather than meeting real ones.

Measuring the value of life

One way around the use of monetary-based techniques has been to start from the value of life or lives. This is seen as fairer and less prone to subjective influence. Decisions as to who should receive services or care are based upon selection criteria drawn up in advance.

Kilner (1990) in his American overview of ethical criteria in patient selection outlines four main types of criteria: social; socio-medical; medical; and personal. His main interest is how these categories interface with the allocation of renal dialysis and transplantable kidneys. Social criteria such as 'social worth' or 'value to society' are regarded as publically unacceptable as they involve overt discrimination against certain social groups, or positive action for favoured groups. Socio-medical criteria such as age, psychological ability and supportive environment are not seen as acceptable in their own right. Denying resources on these criteria alone would be another form of social selection particularly when elderly people are involved; the rule of thumb being – would these people be treated if there was not a scarcity of resources?

Explicit medical criteria need to be based upon the concept of medical-benefit. According to Kilner this method allows treatment to be discontinued if minimum standards of medical benefit are not met. Interestingly, length-of-benefit and quality-of-benefit criteria, which are also connected with this approach but are quantifiable on an index, are regarded as having too high a social price given that patients will already have been assessed on the basis of their ability to benefit from treatment. Such criteria could lead to patients being denied treatment or left to die. Personal Criteria involve among others an ability-to-pay criterion and a random-selection criterion. The first, while widely used in practice, is seen as inherently unfair as an underlying principle; while the second, ironically, is so egalitarian and dependent on chance that it would either result in extra resources or would be suspended.

The valuation of human life in health economics follows very closely the categories outlined above. There are three principle methods of valuing human life:

a) Human Capital approach

b) Willingness to pay approach

c) Quality of Life approach

Each of the above has its own distinct ranking system which more or less overtly contain assumptions about the value of older peoples lives.

Human Capital Approach

Whilst the human capital approach has been rejected by most health economists because of its social unacceptability as an obviously discriminatory device, it is interesting to examine it because it highlights an undercurrent of health economic thought.

The human capital approach values life in terms of the earnings capacity of a person over time. An individual has a stock of health which depreciates over time and the value of that stock is measured in terms of the useful productivity of that person. The analysis can be compared to depreciation policies attached to industrial machinery.

Such an analysis gives little value to the old, the chronically ill and those suffering from a multiplicity of conditions who are usually too ill to participate in any productive process.

Data for valuing human life in the human capital approach is organised around the principle of the individuals remaining productive life years. The value of future life is an area of considerable debate within health economics and demonstrates the influence that value judgements have on the result of the human capital equation. However, what is obvious is that the human capital approach itself has a strong bias against the old, the weak and other economically unproductive members of society. It continually favours those who are economically productive and when ill suffer only a short period of acute illness from which they will soon recover to be productive once more.

The human capital approach is, consequently, an economic measure that reflects the value of productive labour in the market. As such, it perpetuates the inequitable distribution of resources in society and provides the basis for an active discrimination. Avorn makes the point that:'the logic of the human capital argument would thus be perfectly consistent with the concept of euthanasia.' (Avorn 1984, p.1297).

In addition to discriminating against the sick and old the human capital approach introduces a gender bias by valuing women's lives in terms of their lower productive value in the market place. This gender bias is reinforced by the growing proportion of elderly women in society, who under this approach will be even less valued than elderly men.

As pointed out at the beginning of this section, the fact that this method is so obviously discriminatory means that it is generally rejected. However, it is quite easy to see how these ideas are reflected in 'common-sense' notions about resource allocation and which interests are prioritised.

Willingness to Pay Approach

The willingness to pay method measures health care benefits in terms of how much individuals would be willing to spend to avoid or to achieve a particular outcome. Again it is seen as a politically unacceptable method of organising access to health care. Economists, however, find this approach attractive because it is nearest to their concepts of rationality and consumer sovereignty. The concept is based on risk and probability and thus requires a great deal of information for the decision-making process.

The potential of the willingness to pay approach is that it results in valuations derived from individuals' preferences. The method is imprecise, however, because in order to achieve a comparison across different sections of society, weighting must be given to different concepts of risk, different attitudes towards death and disability and differences in economic status. In addition, it is important to identify who is making the decision over willingness to pay and how these decisions are arrived at.

Very often consumers are only able to say that one commodity gives more utility to them than another. They cannot say how much more utility is derived, i.e. they cannot quantify their consumer preference. This is particularly true with respect to health care where quality is difficult to measure and costings are notoriously inaccurate, and the individual's role as consumer is distorted. The problem with this approach, therefore, is that it has a selectivity bias against the elderly and the poor who, relative to the wealthy, the young, and those willing to take risks, may have different concepts of risk and payment. Indeed, differences in economic status can lead to different values in the willingness to pay decision. However, Mishan points out that: 'there is more to be said for rough estimates of the precise concept than precise estimates of economically irrelevant concepts' (Mishan 1971, p.705).

In its defence, the willingness to pay approach has the advantage of attempting to give value of life assessments a social dimension, but an important consideration is that it is still heavily marked by its origins in utilitarian thought and notions of consumer sovereignty. Consequently, it still conceives of the value of life as a commodity with a price that can be traded in the market. In this way, all decisions are only made by people as individuals isolated from society at large. People may make decisions in connection with the health care of others but there is no concept of health care being a social issue. The elderly have no more intrinsic right to health care or a good quality of life in this analysis than in the others. This allows implicit value judgements once again to affect the health care of the elderly. There is no notion of health care as a right – it is merely the result of social altruism. An analysis that depends on the social altruism of others puts the value of life of older people at the mercy of the shifting sands of public opinion.

The relationship between the physician and the individual receiving health care and the difficulties involved with defining health care as an economic good therefore casts doubts over the existence of consumer sovereignty and whether it can be promoted. When health economics gives values to life and health care it is important to question what is being valued and how those values are derived. In this way it may be possible to discover whether the willingness to pay approach is serving the 'consumer' or serving the system.

The danger is all too clear. Health economists who view consumer sovereignty as the rational approach to health care decision-making are forgetting that 'rational choice' does not exist outside the economic and social system itself. By aggregating 'rational choices' health economists are therefore trying to mould the system to their view of it. Put differently, by imposing 'economic rationality' on health care systems health economists are also imposing their definitions of 'rationality' on those systems. Another danger that arises from the willingness to pay approach stems from its dependence on the ability of individuals to fully understand the implications of the decisions they are being asked to make. Can health economists be fully confident that individuals are aware of the consequences of their decisions for their own future and for the future of others?

Nevertheless, what the willingness to pay method does is to introduce a concern with the consequences of health care decisions for other members of society into the equation. It does this by valuing risk in direct and indirect terms (i.e. for the individual and for others). Such a refinement seems to overcome some of the problems associated with other methods of valuing life. It attempts to give value to economically unproductive groups, particularly the elderly and chronically sick. It has the potential to do so through what Culyer (1976) described as the 'caring externality'. This is the result of individuals caring about the health status of others and deriving utility from the provision of such care. The caring externality at present has no place in economic analyses that are concerned with the outcomes of health care, which is after all why we are putting value on life.

Quality Adjusted Life Years

The use of Quality Adjusted Life Years (QALYs) is the most widely known attempt by health economists to intervene in the process of health service decision making. In general it seeks to use generally acceptable socio-medical criteria for rational decision-making in the use of resources. In typical technocratic fashion the originators of the QALY claim to give managers and clinicians a method of making choices by separating 'matters of fact from issues of value'. They assert that they also provide a framework within which the effects of alternative value judgements can be explored (Williams 1989, p.679).

QALYs are based on the axiom that ten years of disability does not have the same value as ten years of good health. Williams states that: 'the essence of a QALY is that it takes a year of healthy life expectancy to be worth one but regards a year of unhealthy life expectancy as worth less than one' (Williams 1985, p.326). It is important to note that the theory gives death a value of nil (0) but that it is possible to be in a state worse than death and thus have a negative value assigned to life.

The index on which these valuations are made is one constructed from patients' own priorities. These are usually gained through the use of questionnaires. The most standardised one (the Rosser Index: see Rosser and Kind 1978) adopts a classification of illness states matrix in which there is a combination of eight degrees of disability and four degrees of distress. These provide 29 categories with which to classify a wide range of health states. Valuations of these health states were gained using a ratio scale rather than an interval one (asking respondents 'how many times more ill is a person in state two than someone in state one?'). The results of these surveys (often using extremely low numbers of respondents) are then aggregated for the purpose of creating QALY tables which can act as a global index for a common scale of measurement (A discussion of these methodologies is contained in Gudex 1986).

A number of problems are associated with this approach. One drawback is the limited number of conditions that the methodology is concerned with. Does only having 29 categories to cover all states of health make the scales less sensitive for certain groups of patients? The work of Donaldson et al (1988), for example, suggests that QALYs are insensitive to the quality-of-life issues of elderly long stay patients. This is especially important when QALYs are being operationalised as ways of making choices between treatment alternatives.

Concern of a more fundamental variety has also been voiced over whether aggregate Quality of Life scores actually represent the opinions and preferences of individuals. This has led one commentator to suggest that 'such research methods do not represent the judgements of individual respondents, but rather create a new reality out of those judgements. Moreover, the analyst's reality can come to be regarded as "more real" than that of the the individuals it is supposed to represent' (quoted in Ashmore, Mulkay and Pinch 1989, p.100). The same commentator also argues that generalizations about patients inclinations are offered by health economists as the attitudes of the patients themselves rather than as the interpretation of the analyst; thus patients are 'willing to sacrifice' a measure of life expectancy for a 'better' quality of life.

That it is the opinion of the analyst that is being put forward is indicated by the importance of what is described as 'constant proportional time trade-off' (Loomes and McKenzie 1989, p.300). This concept is premised on the notion that individuals are prepared to trade some constant proportion of their remaining years of life for a stated improvement in their health, irrespective of how long they are likely to live. However, as Loomes and McKenzie point out, this is only true if the absolute length of time to be spent with less than perfect health (in the case they studied, speech) is more than five years. Consequently, preferences for alternative health scenarios differ greatly with the length of the condition.

In addition, Loomes and McKenzie also point to the importance of the various stages in the life cycle in the determining of time valuation. Good health in middle age may be regarded as more important than that when the individual is young and may fall in late middle age as family responsibilities decrease, only to rise as individuals retire from the workforce. Assessing the evidence they go on to write: 'it suggests that many people may value certain later stages of life more highly than some earlier stages, and therefore adds to the doubts already expressed about the validity of the constant proportional time trade-off assumption' (Loomes and McKenzie 1989, p.301). To this must also be added the actual health of the individual making the valuations. This is particularly important if the individual is suffering from a chronic complaint that has little chance of alleviation, given that their perception of future health states will be influenced by their own present health. This is likely to lead to a divergence in values between acute and chronic forms of illness.

A further difficulty lies at the level of the methodologies used to elicit responses. As is well documented in the literature of survey research, the form in which questions are put can seriously bias the responses (see Bennett and Ritchie 1975). In framing the questions used to construct QALY indexes the hypothetical alternatives posed can have dramatic impact on the resulting valuations as can the use of different methods. Where this happens considerable doubt must be cast on the conclusions and uses to which they are put.

QALYs as Rationing Devices

One of the fundamental principles upon which most advocates of QALYs agree is that QALYs represent a rational method of allocating scarce resources between competing demands on those resources. In viewing them in this fashion their advocates move the terms of debate from the individual to the social. That is, it is no longer a question of utilising QALYs as a way of choosing different forms of treatment for patients on the basis of different combinations of outcomes; rather, it is now a method of ordering these different combinations on the basis of efficiency. It should be remembered that the two previous methods of valuing human life we have examined do not have such all embracing characteristics; possibly one of the reasons for their relative obscurity.

Under the QALY system different combinations of treatment with their different outcomes can now be ranked on the basis of cost. Conditions which are cheap and easy to treat and which have good recovery rates are given greater value in the QALY equation. Similarly, if the cost per QALY of treatment is high then it can be argued that it is not an efficient use of resources. Whether this is a desirable result is open to question, but what is of more importance is that it also allows supposedly objective decisions to be made on the basis of a false legitimacy. It is doubtful whether any group of respondents from which the QALY indexes were constructed would agree to their valuations being used as the basis of denying resources to certain groups (and it is highly unlikely that they were told about this dimension of their answers).

The social dimension of the use of QALYs raises other questions too. An important one is weighting; that is the procedures used to ensure that particular groups (such as elderly people) are not discriminated against by the processes of economic evaluation. Weightings are essential under any system of rationing if equity is to be maintained. Under the QALY system older people are most at risk because of the imbalance that can be put on the idea of an extra year of healthy life at 70 compared with that at 40. Making individuals' valuations the basis of an aggregate cannot but discriminate against older people (Gudex 1986). Because such discrimination is deemed illegitimate if equity is to be maintained, the QALY system cannot say anything conclusive about the appropriate weightings necessary for older people. This again leaves the decisions in the hands of the health economists who have an interest in giving periods of bad health lower values in order to make their models work. So, far from removing value judgements from allocative decision-making, the QALY system concentrates it in fewer 'value free' hands.

This reflects what Harris (1987) argues is the weakness of QALYs: that they value years rather than peoples lives. As a result there is a bias towards the young and against elderly people. A more serious danger lies in what Harris refers to as 'Double Jeopardy'. He explains it in the following terms:

> QALYs dictate that once an individual is unfortunate, because he or she has once become a victim of disaster, we are required to visit upon him or her a second and perhaps graver misfortune…The first disaster leaves the patient with a poor quality of life and QALYs require that because of this, he or she be ruled out as a candidate for life saving treatment, or at best that he or she be given little or no chance of benefiting from what little amelioration the condition allows. (Harris 1987, p.108)

The use of QALYs by managers and clinicians is clearly open to misuse as a way of preventing resources from being channelled to the elderly and chronically sick. They can therefore become what Harris calls 'a life threatening device'. One way of using such a device is to switch patients with low QALYs from life-saving care to life-enhancing care, by providing a socially acceptable minimum of care. One example of this would be to place the chronically sick in voluntary funded hospices for the terminally ill thereby removing from the health service the need to pay for or provide costly acute services to this group. Another example is the movement towards active euthanasia in Holland and the pressures on the elderly that this entails (see Fenigsen 1989).

However, there is another need to address in looking at the impact of the QALY system; namely that of its methodological individualism. This makes itself clearest in QALYs inability to address distributional issues. As Loomes and McKenzie (1989) point out, cost-per-QALY rankings are not concerned with the distribution of QALYs between individuals, but only with the total numbers of QALYs that can be generated by a given input of resources. Consequently, the issue of social welfare is of a minor importance.

That this is a particular problem can be seen when the issue of universal free health care is approached. The motivation for such a system did not come from the perceived efficiency gains that such a system would procure, rather, it came from a desire to provide the maximum possible health care to all of the population. It was not based on a notion of setting limits to availability of health care and still isn't. By trying to base a system of resource allocation on 'timeless' individual opinions about abstract health care scenarios the advocates of QALYs miss much of the point of public attitudes towards issues of health care. It could be argued that their agenda is as much a political one as it is economic. Klein (1989) points out that there is more than one (economic) rationality in the field of health care resource allocation. This point needs to be constantly re-emphasised.

To summarise, all methods of valuing human life for planning purposes discriminate unfairly against older people. Going back for a moment to Kilner's (1990) categories of patient selection criteria we can see that the methods of evaluation used by health economists all fall within categories that Kilner sees as unacceptable. The human capital approach is essentially a social criterion and as such involves judgements of worth derived from economic potential. These are not necessarily generally accepted by the population at large and are inherently unfair. The willingness-to-pay approach is based upon a personal criterion which exaggerates the inequalities already present in society to greater levels and must therefore involve the creation of a less equitable health care system. The QALY method, although involving medical criteria, is still a system of social rationing; a socio-medical criterion to use Kilner's term. None of the methods outlined use purely medical criteria and it is probably for this reason that they have become contentious.

It is important to recognise that health economics as a discipline is probably faced with an impossible task when it tries to find acceptable social bases for restricting budgets (or for choosing between different financial options). However, in maintaining that such an objective is possible, utilisers of the tools of health economics are guilty of perpetuating myths that can cloak discrimination.

Health Economics, Moral Panics and Social Policy

In this chapter we have attempted to outline how the methods of mainstream health economics contain implicit assumptions and unstated conclusions about older people. These ideas do not exist in a vacuum. Concern about the 'greying of the population' is widespread throughout the industrialised world. The American health care system is seen by many to be challenged by a growing population of elderly dependent individuals, who are likely to consume growing levels of financial resources. This has prompted some analysts to talk about an intergenerational crisis. While this frightening scenario may be limited to the fringes of political life in America, our discussion suggests that, in the ideas of health economics, it is one that has broader echoes. This extends to the way in which health economists explicitly deal with the needs of elderly people. As an example of this, two health economists – Scitovsky and Capron (1986) point to the high medical expenses of the elderly in relation to other sections of the population. They write:

> A very large share of the elderly's medical care expenditures are incurred in the last year or even months of their lives; this has led to the question of whether scarce resources are being 'wasted' on the dying, resources that could be spent more productively on other patients.' (Scitovsky and Capron 1986, p.60)

Correspondingly, they argue that high medical expenses are being expended at the end of life on care 'of very ill but not necessarily dying patients'. This is a value judgement on the social worth of these individuals. Scitovsky and Capron speculate that it will be with this group of patients that physicians and economists will face the ethical dilemma of demographic change. Callahan sees the growing elderly population as 'a new social threat' and argues that as a result: 'Medicine should be used not for the further expansion of the life of the aged, but for the full achievement of a natural and fitting life span and thereafter for the relief of suffering'. (Callahan 1987, p.53)

Such views prompted by the ideas of health economics can only bring pressure to bear on clinical practices and may lead to a real setting of limits to care. Thomasma noted this tendency to put the health care needs of the elderly into a separate category when he wrote:

> Some proposals to allocate health care on the basis of age seem to move the elderly into the house of the dead, precisely because they 'cut off' the elderly from the modes of care we offer to other persons in society. (Thomasma 1989, p.170)

Enormous pressures are being brought to bear on the elderly in the form of appeals for them to cut their demand for health care so that the young can benefit more. Indeed Churchill argues that: 'Such a gesture should not appear to us as a sacrifice, but as the ordinary virtue entailed by a just, social conscience' (Churchill 1988, p.647).

These conclusions are not the product of historial accident. Estes (1989) outlines the ideological aspects of cost containment policies to show that one of the major consequences of laissez-faire economics for health care was a shift in responsibility from corporate bodies to the individual. Older people, according to this developing ideology, have got to take more responsibility for their health and well-being. And those who don't are perceived as an economic and social burden. Interestingly, recent UK government policy on pensions (abolition of State Earnings Related Supplement – SERPS) and private health insurance for elderly people (making it tax-deductible) are indications of this approach. Here, once again, the echoes of the neo-classical economic notion of productive worth are all too apparent.

Conclusion

The importance of utilitarianism for health economics cannot be underestimated. Indeed, the concept of utility derived from health care has been discussed at length in this paper. In their efforts to quantify the utility of different types of health care so that resources can be allocated on the basis of that utility, economists are by-passing another important idea, namely the right to health care. Health economists must reassess their role in determining the allocation of resources and look at methods of efficiently directing resources so that no group is denied health care by default.

The real irony of arguments that try to justify a cut-off for different forms of treatment on the basis of age and cost is that they ignore the individual needs, at the same time as demanding individual sacrifice because of the scarcities within the public sector. Hilfiker (1983) argued that limits to care already exist in physician behaviour and that the old, the chronically ill, and the mentally ill do not receive the same levels of aggressive treatment as the young acutely ill.

The existence of such unofficial rationing policies should be a major cause for concern. Instead, what seems to be happening is that economic arguments are being used to support and strengthen such policies. Policies that many health economists would not accept are being promoted because some clinicians and health care managers are using health economics as a tool and not as a discipline. Clinicians are doing this oblivious of the tendency of health economics to present itself in terms of laissez-faire and utilitarian approaches, approaches which ignore the importance of any social welfare function.

If, in the current period of financial stringency, one imagines acute health services taking on the form of a sieve, then there is a growing predisposition to make the holes in that sieve bigger so that more and more people slip through. If the size of the holes is being determined by clinical considerations then care is being limited on the basis of providing health care to as many people as possible as well as preventing unnecessary pain and suffering. If however the size of the holes is being influenced by cost then questions of resource allocation and opportunity cost may be the main considerations being addressed. If the size of the holes is being determined by ageist policies coupled with calls for cost containment then there is a danger that the system is becoming morally bankrupt.

Health economics needs to be a discipline that makes clear to clinicians the problems of resource allocation and the concept of opportunity cost. What it must not become is a tool of those who are arguing for cost containment on the basis of age, race, gender or social class. The danger of this occurring is considerable if the assumptions and the value judgements that form the basis of economic analysis are not made explicit. Economists must develop new measures that incorporate distributional issues into social welfare functions before measures are applied to health care. These need to stress the rights of all individuals to health care, whatever their age or background. They also need to incorporate non-discriminatory objectives that bring out the best in a universalist health care system and not its worst technocratic tendencies. Above all, what needs to be achieved is an awareness, among those involved in making decisions, of the consequences of their ideas and actions.

Notes

1. Macroeconomics: '…deals with the behaviour of the economy as a whole – or with the broad aggregates of economic life. It is the study of the overall level of a nation's output, employment, unemployment and prices'. Samuelson and Nordhaus 1985, p.77.
2. Utilitarianism: Economics is the study of choice; that is choices made under conditions of scarcity. At the centre of this discipline lies the philosophy of utilitarianism which sees the maximisation of social utility as axiomatic.

The relevance of utilitarianism to health care has been questioned by writers such as Veatch (1980) who argue that utilitarianism allows subgroups within a society to be excluded from the allocation of scarce resources if the society as a whole benefits.

Health economists have countered that such arguments deal with 'vulgar' utilitarianism and ignore sophistications that address process utility and the caring externality. With respect to health care, however, utilitarianism is still open to the criticism that it can lead to individuals being denied care: a) through the precedence given to the 'common good'; and b) because of a lack of adequate information on who benefits from different allocative scenarios.

Health economics and the utilitarianism on which it is based can therefore be criticised on theoretical and technical grounds. Whilst it may indeed provide a 'rational' alternative to exisitng allocative decision making, there are alternatives to the utilitarian tradition such as theories of need, justice and ethics which can and do provide alternatives of their own whilst addressing the weaknesses of the utilitarian model.

References

Ashmore, M., Mulkay, M., and Pinch, T. (1989) *Health and Efficiency: A Sociology of Health Economics.* Milton Keynes: Open University Press.

Avorn, J. (1984) Benefits and Cost analysis in Geriatric Care. *The New England Journal of Medicine* 310 (20) 1294-1301.

Bennett, A., and Ritchie, K., (1975) *Questionnaires in Medicine: A quide to their design and use.* Oxford: Nuffield Provincial Hospitals Trust/Oxford University Press.

Brooks, R. (1985) *Efficiency in health care. In Long, A. and Harrison, S. eds Health Service Performance – Effectiveness and Efficiency*, 57–80. London: Croom Helm.

Callahan, D. (1987) *Setting Limits, Medical Goals in an Ageing Society.* New York: Simon and Schuster.

Churchill, L. R. (1986) Should we ration health care by age? *Journal of the American Geriatrics Society* 36 (7) 644-647.

Culyer, A. J. (1976) *Need and the National Health Service.* London: Martin Robertson.

Donaldson, C., Atkinson, A., Bond, J., Wright, K., (1988). QALYs and long-term care for elderly people in the UK: scales for assessment of quality of life. *Age and Ageing* 17, 379-387.

Estes, C., (1989) Cost containment and the elderly, Conflict or challenge? *Journal of the American Geriatrics Society* 36 (1) 68-72.

Evans, J. G., (1990) Symposium. The ethics of resource allocation. *Journal of Epidemiology and Community Health* 44, 187- 190.

Fenigsen, R., (1989) A case against Dutch euthanasia, Special Supplement. *Hastings Centre Report*, January/February, 1-16.

Gudex, C., (1986) QALYs and their use by the Health Service. *Discussion paper 20.* University of York Centre for Health Economics.

Harris, J., (1988) Equality. In Brune, P. (ed) *Health Rights and Resources.* Kings College Studies 1987-88.

Hilfiker, A., (1983) Allowing the debilitated to die. *New England Journal of Medicine* 308, 716.

Johnson, P., Conrad, E., and Thomson. D., (eds) (1989) *Workers Versus Pensioners.* Manchester: Manchester University Press.

Kilner, J. F., (1990) *Who Lives? Who Dies? Ethical criteria in patient selection.* Boston: Yale University Press.

Klein, R., (1989) The Role of Health Economics. *British Medical Journal* 299, 275-276.

Loomes, G., McKenzie, L., (1989) The use of QALYs in Health Care decision making. *Social Science and Medicine* 28 (4) 299-308.

Maynard, A., (1990) Symposium. The ethics of resource allocation. *Journal of Epidemiology and Community Health* 44, 187-190.

McGuire, A., Henderson J., and Mooney, G., (1989) *The economics of Health Care.* London: Routledge and Kegan Paul.

Mishan, E. J., (1971) Evaluation of Life and Limb, A Theoretical approach. *Journal of Political Economy* 79 (4) July / August 687-705.

Mooney, G. H., (1983) *Economics, Medicine and Health Care.* Hassocks: Wheatsheaf.

NHS Management Inquiry (1983): *Report.* London: DHSS (Griffiths Report).

Rosser, R., Kind, P., (1978) A scale of valuation of states of illness: is there a social consensus? *International Journal of Epidemiology* 7, 347-357.

Samuelson, P. A., Nordhaus (1985) *Economics. 12th Edition,* p.950. New York: McGraw-Hill Book Company.

Schwartz, D., Reilly, P., (1986) The choice not to be resuscitated. *Journal of the American Geriatrics Society* 34, 807.

Scitovsky, A. A., Capron, A. M., (1986) Medical Care at the end of life: the interaction of economics and ethics. *Annual Review of Public Health* 7, 59-75.

Thomasma, D. C., (1987) Moving the aged into the house of the dead. *Journal of the American Geriatrics Society* 37 (2) 169-172 .

Williams, A., (1985) Economics of coronary artery bypass grafting. *British Medical Journal* 291, 326-329.

Williams, A., (1989) The Role of Health Economic (letter). *British Medical Journal* 299, 679.

Working for Patients (1989) Department of Health: HMSO.

Veatch, R. M., (1980) *A Theory of Medical Ethics.* New York: Basic Books.

CHAPTER 9

Policy Development at the Grassroots Level

Silvana di Gregorio

This chapter is very much about ideas-in-progress as well as work-in-progress. The ideas begin with a consideration of the nature of social policy, the nature of research and their inter-relationship. The work is based on a project called the Age Exchange in Bedfordshire, England, which has set up five independent forums throughout the county which bring together service providers who cater for older people from the statutory, voluntary and private sectors. Age Exchange provides a vehicle through which to explore the possibilities of facilitating 'bottom-up' policy making, or policy development at the grassroots level.

Social Policy and Research

The ideas for this study began in the early 1980s when I was concerned that three-quarters of research on older people in Britain involved policy and practice and most of it had been commissioned by central government departments (Todd and Taylor 1981), particularly the then Department of Health and Social Security (DHSS). (This single Department has since been divided into the Department of Health (DoH), and the Department of Social Security (DSS)). As a sociologist, I was interested in the influences on the development of social gerontology, and had traced the dominance of social policy 'concerns of the moment' within this evolving discipline (di Gregorio 1986). There was little work on developing the theoretical side of the discipline, hence theory was not informing the direction of research. However, while social policy concerns seemed to be shaping the ways old age was being researched, very little of the findings from this research was being used to alter practice (Illsley 1983). The situation, then, could be summarised as follows:

- government departments were setting the agenda of issues for the study of old age (social gerontology);
- in order to get funding for projects researchers accepted this agenda while (for the most part) recognising the limitations this placed for developing their discipline;

- most findings never reached practitioners or local policy makers; and
- in a general review of DHSS funded projects by the Department and sponsored researchers, it was agreed that there was no mechanism to translate policy findings into local contextual needs.

There are a number of questions raised by this situation. For example, who should set the agenda of issues for the study of old age? What are the appropriate roles for government departments, researchers and practitioners? Are government departments to set policy, researchers to find facts and practitioners to receive facts? Is the way forward to ensure proper lines of communication between central government departments and local policy-makers?

Donald Schon (1971) has pointed out that the prevailing theory of (what he calls) 'public learning': 'is that the formation and implementation of public policy is a rational process which takes place in the centre-periphery mode.' Challis *et al* (1988) have identified this tradition of public policy and rationality in Britain. In brief, there is:

1. an emphasis on basing decisions on the analysis of information;
2. an identification of rationality with adopting a systematic, holistic view of any given problem;
3. a reliance on technique and machinery for problem solving;
4. a strong preoccupation with the organisational structure of policy making; and
5. a stress on the key role of coordination as an instrument of rationality.

But both Challis *et al* and Schon have shown that this rational approach to policy making is in itself irrational. It ignores the inherent conflict between central and local policymakers. The former see local policies as not taking account of developments elsewhere and possibly also conflicting with its own policy line. Those at the local level see central policymakers as out of touch with the realities of their situation and find policies coming from above as unworkable.

However, the traditional reason for explaining why policies are not being carried out is the lack of coordination. Better coordination is held out as the key for ensuring proper policy implementation. But this 'rational' response is still not responding to the fact that often central policies do not fit local needs.

Part of the reason for this mismatch of needs is that social policies are complex. Policies for older people, for example, cut across government departments. Department of Health for health services, Department of Social Security for personal social services and income maintenance etc. At the local level, this is further complicated by whatever voluntary services are operating in an area, local transport policies, local educational opportunities for older people as well as local provision from the private sector. In

Britain there is no established agency which contains all the elements to act upon a comprehensive policy for older people. Yet the 'rational approach' to policymaking acts as though there is.

The 'rational approach' also assumes that policymaking is apolitical. That 'experts' will collect neutral facts from which policies depicting self-evident values can be constructed. Phillipson and Walker (1987) have argued that much of social gerontology is based on a false positivism, and reflects the false assumption that the establishment of scientific facts is distinct from proposals of what to do with them. They propose a more value-committed approach to social gerontology – one which would not just aim to *understand* the social construction of ageing but one which would also aim to *change* it.

Challis *et al* (1988) show how the Thatcher years in Britain have exposed the reality once and for all, that the ends of social policy are often political. For the Thatcher government, policy analysis was clearly the servant of politics rather than an independent source of ideas and policies. Coordination of policies, instead of being seen as a tool of rationality, in this light can be seen as a tool of coercion.

Given the complexity of social problems, Schon (1971) claims that a centre-periphery approach to policymaking cannot work as it depends on giving a stable, relatively simple message which can be spread uniformly over a periphery. Instead, he advocates a new model for policymaking, shift away from the centre-periphery model to one which centres on network modes of growth and diffusion.

By focusing on building policy from the local level, Schon is addressing the mismatch between local needs and central policy. Schon does not see the role of central government as first seeking the correct solution to a problem, then training society in its adaptation. Instead he sees the periphery or the local area as the location where solutions to problems are being worked out. He sees the role of central government as:

> detect(ing) significant changes at the periphery,...pay(ing) explicit attention to the emergence of ideas in good currency, and...deriv(ing) themes of policy by induction...Central (government) comes to function as a facilitator of society's learning, rather than as society's trainer. (p.177)

While Schon's ideas are attractive as a solution to devising policies to fit local needs, they still ignore the political dimension of the ends of any social policy. And given the current political climate in Britain, where one can see central government as taking on the role of 'society's trainer', there are limits to which one can apply Schon's ideas, anyway. However, his use of networks to develop local policies is relevant. This has a lot to do with the loose conceptualisation around current 'buzz words' such as networks, interagency collaboration etc. They are part of the language of central government policymakers. For them, however, 'networks', 'coordination' and 'collaboration' are seen as instruments to ensure the implementation of their central political aims for social policy. However, given the currency of such ideas, there does not seem to be any obstacles to develop policy from networks – as Schon suggests.

Informal networks crop up wherever no established agency exists to tackle a 'whole problem' – such as community care for older people. Schon argues that such informal networks serve as a kind of 'shadow system' which can form the basis for developing a real system – for community care in this instance.

However, one needs to understand the political dimension of any such 'shadow system'. Challis *et al* (1988), in looking at inter-agency collaboration, found that those who stood to gain from successful outcomes of coordination were a diffuse and unorganised constituency. Those who stood to gain from the maintenance of the status quo are by definition concentrated and organised. However, they did find examples of successful collaboration. Such collaboration occurred where there was a strong value predisposition towards system-wide thinking and where there were prolonged opportunities for interaction across boundaries to permit learning about different practices and to develop trust. Other incentives were also needed – including powerful representation of the client's interests and needs, and resource incentives.

So what is the role of research in developing this form of grassroots policymaking? I mentioned earlier Phillipson and Walker's plea for a more value-committed social gerontology. They mention a need to provide new approaches to the continuing education of health and social care professionals. I see the facilitating of 'shadow networks' of service provision for older people as a small step in that direction. Research has a role to play in this facilitation, not as a tool in the hands of some 'detached' expert, but rather as a tool to be used by the participants of these 'shadow networks'. This is putting the locus of control of research in the hands of professionals and service providers.

Research in the Hands of Service Providers?

People with professional experience working in a local area know all too well the limits of their practice. It is after all those professionals in daily contact with older people who make public policy in the routines they establish and the ways they cope with the pressures of work. Given the tools of research they can be made more reflective of their practice. However, reflection alone may not be enough to ensure a better social construction of old age. In fact, it could perpetuate an image of frailty and dependency in later life. If that is, research is left to those professionals whose training has been dominated by a pathology model of ageing. However, if we broaden the notion of service providers for older people to include adult educators and librarians, for example, the interaction between this varied mix of professionals could lead to the incorporation of a more balanced view of older people – one which includes the positive images of an active later life.

The Age Exchange project brings together this mix of providers and introduces them to the tools of research and to the possibility of bottom-up policymaking.

The Project

The Age Exchange project has five forums which cover the county of Bedfordshire. These forums are based in Luton, Dunstable, Leighton Buzzard, Mid-Bedfordshire and Bedford, and bring together service providers who cater for older people from the statutory, voluntary and private sectors. Membership of the forums is voluntary and attracts those service providers who place a high value on inter-agency collaboration. At the time of writing there were about 150 members of the Age Exchange county-wide.

The first stage in developing this project was to endorse the idea of the Age Exchange in Bedfordshire. Those who were initially responsible for enabling the Age Exchange project to develop had their own reasons for sponsoring it. The initiative came from joint finance trainers who wanted an opportunity to bring together service providers, particularly from the voluntary sector county-wide, to help people begin to think about working together. Bedfordshire had just set up a Joint Care Planning Team (JCPT; 'Joint' i.e.between Health and Social Service providers) to produce a strategic framework for service provision for older people up to the turn of the century. One of the originating trainers was on this team and saw the forums as a way of reaching the voluntary sector and make sure that they would find the JCPT's proposals acceptable. In other words, she (the trainer) saw the Age Exchange as a way to facilitate the implementation of a top-down policy initiative – rather than endorse grassroots policymaking.

We first agreed to hold a study day which would promote working together between the statutory, voluntary and private sectors. The initial thinking of the JCPT on elderly people would be presented. In addition, the Age Exchange idea would be introduced. It would be left to the participants of the meeting whether they would want to develop the Age Exchange forums in their area. In the event, the meeting enthusiastically endorsed the Age Exchange idea. Liaison Officers for each area were nominated and the scene was set for developing the forums. The professionals and service providers had responded to the opportunity of extending their networks with other service providers, identifying 'good practice' and understanding the needs of the client group. The idea that they could have a say in policymaking was a very new one and most of them did not see it as a possibility.

The second stage of the project was to establish the membership of the five forums. Liaison Officers for the five areas had been nominated during the Age Exchange study day. Their job together with the Development

Officer was to ensure that the forum included as wide a representation as possible of representatives from all the organisations which had anything to do with older people in the area. They also attempted to have a balance between managers and practitioners.

The agencies and professional groups who were invited to attend the first Leighton Buzzard forum meeting in June 1988 are listed in Table 9.1. At that meeting they were asked which groups they felt were missing from the forum. The resulting list of missing agencies is shown in Table 9.2.

Table 9.1. Agencies invited to first Leighton Buzzard forum meeting

DHSS	*Local Information Officer**
Education	SALP – Special Adult Learning Programme*
Health	Community Occupational Therapist
	Community Psychiatric Nurse*
	District Nursing Sister*
	General Practitioner
	Health Care Manager*
Housing	Housing Management Officer*
	Sheltered Housing Warden*
	Private Sector Representative*
Social Services	Domiciliary Care Organizer*
	Elderly and Handicap Team – Section Manager*
	Organiser, Social Centre
	Social Worker*
Voluntary	Carers Help and Support Group*
	Carers Self-Help Group
	Council of Churches
	Council of Voluntary Organiaztions*
	Retirement Group
	Senior Citizens Association*
	Tenant Representative of Sheltered Housing*
	WRVS, District Organizer

* invited and attended

In this way the membership of the forums was extended. However, this method relies on bringing together already existing networks. Certain agencies remain outside this network – particularly regarding services provided by the different ethnic communities. In Leighton Buzzard, for example, there are Polish and Italian communities. In Bedford and Luton, there are also Asian and Afro-Caribbean communities. The forum members had virtually no links with these communities and it became obvious that more outreach work would need to be done to establish contacts. This became one of the tasks of the forums which I will expand upon below.

Table 9.2 Leighton Buzzard forum: missing agencies and groups

Church	
Health	General Practitioners Health Visitors Pharmacists
Library	
Police	
Social Services	Home Helps Occupational Therapists Social Centre Westlands Residential Home (local)
Voluntary	Women's Royal Voluntary Service (WRVS) Senior Citizens Association Retirement Association Citizens Advice Bureau St. John's Ambulance Befrienders National Association for the Care and Resettlement of Offenders (NACRO) Local Victim Support Group
Users/Carers	

The third stage of the project was to make attending the forums a worthwhile experience. Some forum members were accustomed to attending committee style meetings which discussed cooperation between agencies but got nowhere. They were anxious that the forums would amount to just 'talking shops'. There was quite a bit of underlying scepticism during the first couple of forum meetings.

This period of scepticism (which was experienced by some forums more acutely than others) reached a peak by the time of the second or third forum meeting. It was during this time that the membership of the forums was being established. Part of the confusion was due to the problems of incorporating new members. All the forums had a core of members who had attended the original study day and were committed to the idea that the forums had an important educative function. This educative aspect of the forums – that members could learn from one another – was something which some of the newer members were slow to pick up. (Many initially asserted that they knew everything about local services.) Another part of the confusion was that in some areas where a number of different old people's organisations were competing with one another, the forum was seen as another competitor which was doing something that they should be doing. These difficulties receded into the background when the forum members could begin to see the results of the tasks that they had set.

So the fourth turning point for the project was the articulation of the tasks of the forum. From the very beginning the forums were task-centred. The first task of all the forums was an information gathering exercise on all local provision which may be of interest to older people. Initially this was conceived as a local resource book on 'good practice'. Although many of the professionals in the forums were keen on identifying 'good practice' right away, I managed to persuade them that a definition of 'good practice' was something which forum members would have to slowly evolve together. However, none of the forum areas had any comprehensive directory of services for older people. One of the forums proposed that the information on the services should be used to produce a consumer booklet. This booklet would be more than just a directory, it would give the consumer more information on the background of the schemes in order to put the service into context. In this way each consumer could decide whether the service is for them. All the forums agreed to this proposal.

Specifically, it was agreed that the information gathering would be carried out by retired people who would visit each scheme and interview the appropriate manager or organiser responsible for it. In addition to collecting information for the booklets, they would be asking detailed questions on staffing, funding, links each organisation had with others and links they would like to develop as well as how they saw the service developing in the future. This information would provide the forum with some of the raw material with which to consider policy development. Many members were very keen to consider gaps and overlaps in service provision, but at this stage they could not see how they could have an impact on policy.

The fifth and sixth stages of the project were about forum members learning to set their own agendas and beginning to take control of the forums – this is the stage the forums have reached to date. It has been marked by a gradual realisation by forum members that they may have a role to play in the development of policy. As I mentioned earlier, in extending the membership of the forums, members were struck forcibly by the fact that they had hardly any links with the ethnic communities. Forum members are now beginning to do something about that. The Bedford forum is starting to build links with members of its ethnic communities. This process has had the added benefit of uncovering links with the ethnic communities in Luton. Very little is known about what services these communities provide for ethnic elders. What is known is that current statutory and voluntary services do not cater for their needs.

The forums have also identified that the provision of transport is one of the biggest problems in the county. A Dial-a-Ride scheme run by a voluntary organisation operates in the south of the county. The organiser of that scheme, who is a forum member, proposed that the Age Exchange call a county-wide meeting of representatives from all the forums together with relevant transport people from County Hall and the National Advisory Unit on Transport to consider the problem. In addition, forum members are considering ways of distributing the consumer booklet to ensure it gets to the widest possible audience. They are also beginning to think of other ways to disseminate information.

These three issues – links with ethnic communities, transport and dissemination of information – are all being considered by separate sub-groups of each forum. This gives forum members a responsibility for a particular area of policy and encourages sub-groups to get together on a county-wide basis to consider these problems. Forum members are taking on more and more responsibility for the work of the forums.

The final stage of the project is for the forums to be actually involved in policymaking. The Joint Consultative Committee's (JCCs)[1] Strategic Framework for Elderly People of Bedfordshire 1989–2001, seems to be acting as a trigger to enable this to happen. It had been agreed from the beginning of the project that the forums would be used as part of the consultative mechanism once the Strategic Framework was produced.

In a way it was fortuitous that the JCC would consult the forums on what was basically a top-down policy document which in effect would be anticipating the government's response to the Griffiths Report[2]. Professionals welcomed the opportunity to be part of the consultation process; in their own organisations such a document would not filter down to them. In fact, when the document finally came out in May 1989 it did not filter down to most professionals and service providers. For most of them, being in a position to respond to a policy document was a new role. It has encouraged them to reflect on their own values. It has also started them to develop policies of their own.

How far the forums will be able to make an impact on transport policy in the county, or on policies sensitive to the needs of ethnic communities and the older consumer remains to be seen. But the forums are beginning to engage in policymaking through the development of what Schon would call their 'shadow networks'.

Addendum

The Age Exchange was one of only a handful of organisations which sent to the JCC a detailed response to their Strategic Framework for Services for Older People. A year after sending in the response, the Age Exchange received the Final Version of the Strategic Framework. This document, apart from a few minor changes, was substantially the same as the document that went out for consultation. Most of the points made in the Age Exchange's response were ignored.

On a more positive note, the forums have been making a significant impact on transport policy in the county. The county-wide meeting on transport was a success and was followed by a series of meetings devoted to transport in each of the five forums. These were attended by the Community Transport Officer from Bedfordshire County Council who was keen

Table 9.3 Age Exchange Bedfordshire – Turning points

August 1987	Meeting to consider a study day to promote an exchange of knowledge of services for older people in the County of Bedfordshire
March 1988	County-wide study day Launch of the Age Exchange Liaison Officers from different areas nominated
April 1988	Appointment of Development Officer
May-Aug 1988	Setting up of 5 forums
Sept-Dec 1988	Extending/establishing forum membership Refining aims; roles of members Mini-crises on aims of forum Beginning to collate list of services for older people
January 1988	Development Officer left Sharpening of aims
Feb-March 1989	Training first information gatherers (two forums) Finalising list of schemes to be visited
April 1989	New Development Officer appointed Half-time Administrator appointed Information Gathering begins
May-July 1989	JCC Strategic Framework for Services for Older People produced Hold consultation meetings on the document with each forum Identify policy needs of forums transport links with ethnic communities Discussion of form of disseminating information of schemes to consumers Establish sub-groups within each forum to take more responsibility for forum work Information gathering continues Training of more information gatherers
August 1989	Production of Age Exchange Response to Strategic Framework Training of more information gatherers Information gathering continues
Sept-Dec 1989	Forum Meetings on developing policy County-wide sub-group meetings transport ethnic communities format of consumer booklet Links with Bedfordshire and Buckinghamshire Information Service

Jan-Apr 1990	Individual forum meetings on transport policy Developing data base format for services Information gathering continues Sub-groups begin to extract data from the questionnaires Begin planning of distribution and media launch of booklet
May-Oct 1990	Decision to go ahead with booklets in 3 of the 5 forum areas Decision to concentrate on transport policy and other policy issues in other 2 areas Realise that booklets are really books (Bedford book is 144 pages) Continue with extraction of data from questionnaires Finalise form of entry Sub-groups work on distribution of books and organising local services fair to launch book Discuss design of book with printer (one area sets a competition among older people in the area to design the cover of the book) Input data extracted from questionnaires onto computer data base Final edit of Bedford book Discussions with interested parties from Age Concern England and Help the Aged about future of forums
Nov 1990	Launch of Age Matters: A consumer's guide to services in North Bedfordshire Organise Age Matters Fair – on local services and opportunities for older people in North Bedfordshire
Jan-June 1991	Launch of Age Matters: A consumer's guide to services in Mid-Bedfordshire Age Exchange forums to become independent of Cranfield Second phase—looking at data on services, identifying gaps/overlaps, looking at feedback from consumers on services, developing local policies, acting as an agency for advocacy, begin update on consumer book

to consult local groups on transport policy. The result has been a new Dial-a-Ride service in the north of the county, an improved Dial-a-Ride service in the south of the county and other community bus services in the pipeline.

The production of consumer guides has occupied most of the time of the forums during 1990. Members of the forums were fully involved in analysing the information collected on services for older people and in deciding on what information should be covered in the consumer guide. The first book on services for older people in North Bedfordshire was launched in November 1990 and was instantly a success. There are 120 schemes covered in the book. A Consumer guide for Mid-Bedfordshire was published in June 1991.

The action-research phase of this project is now almost over. Negotiations are being made to ensure that the forums will be self-managing by the end of 1991. Table 9.3 indicates the major turning points of this project.

Notes

1. Joint Consultative Committees (JCC) were set up following the reorganisation of the National Health Service in Britain in 1974, in recognition of the large degree of overlap which existed between the health and welfare services. District Health Authorities and Local Authorities are required to set up JCCs of their members to review and coordinate plans and to advise on the operation of the two services. Since 1984 there has been a statutory duty in Regional Health Authorities to appoint additional members to the JCC from the voluntary sector.

   The Bedfordshire JCC acknowledged that it had few links with the voluntary sector in the county and knew little of the services they provided. Some members of the JCC saw the Age Exchange forums as a ready-made network into the voluntary sector which they could use to make known to that sector how they wish to make use of their services. Although the Strategic Framework claimed to be consultative, in practice it was more of a top-down policy document.
2. Sir Roy Griffiths was asked by the then Secretary of State for Social Services, Mr Norman Fowler, to undertake an overview of community care policy on 16th December 1986. The terms of reference were:

   > to review the way in which public funds are used to support community care policy and to advise me on options which would improve the use of these funds as a contribution to more effective community care.

   The Griffiths Report which came out in March 1988 concentrated on adults who require care and support because they are elderly, mentally ill, mentally handicapped or physically disabled. It encompassed the roles of families and friends; volunteers and the organised voluntary sector; private profit making services; and public services in the provision of community care. The Report focused on the action needed in the fields of personal social services, health services and social security. It recommended that local authority social service departments would take the lead in consulting with the National Health Service, the voluntary, and the private sectors in coming up with local community care plans. They would also be responsible for assessing individual's needs for support in the home and the design of individual packages of care. This would enable them to take a comprehensive view of community care.

The Government did not respond to the Report until November 1989 when it published the White Paper on Community Care, Caring for People (Cm. 849, 1989). The full implementation of the resulting NHS and Community Care Act 1990 has been delayed until April 1993. This is the last of a succession of major pieces of social legislation which have major implications for the reduction of power of the local authorities and the change from local authorities being the main providers of social welfare to being contractors of welfare from external agencies. (The other pieces of legislation are the Education Reform Act, 1988; the Housing Act, 1988; and the Local Government Finance Act, 1988.)

The JCC, recognising that the Griffiths Report could have major implications for the management of community care, decided to produce a number of 'strategic frameworks' for the different client groups affected by community care. Bedfordshire had few links with the voluntary or private sectors so it seems likely they wanted to ensure a favourable reception to their ideas before being forced to change by the government.

References

Challis, L., Fuller, S., Klein, R., Henwood, M., Plowden, W., Webb, A., Whittingham, P. and Wistow, G. (1988) *Joint Approaches to Social Policy: Rationality and Practice.* Cambridge University Press.

di Gregorio, S. (1986) *Growing Old in Twentieth Century Leeds: An exploratory study based on the life histories of people aged 75 years and over, with specific reference to their past and present management of everyday living – at home and at work.* Unpublished PhD thesis, LSE University of London.

Griffiths, R. (1988) *Community Care: Agenda for Action* London: HMSO

Illsley, R. (1983) 'The Contribution of Research to the Development of Practice and Policy'. In *DHSS Research Contribution to the Development of Policy and Practice.* London: HMSO.

Phillipson, C. and Walker, A. (1987) 'The Case for a Critical Gerontology.' In di Gregorio, S. (ed) *Social Gerontology: New Directions.* London: Croom Helm.

Schon, D. (1971) *Beyond the Stable State.* London: Temple Smith.

Todd, H. and Taylor, H. (1981) *Social Gerontology in Britain: From Research to Policy.* Paper presented at XII International Congress of Gerontology, Hamburg.

CHAPTER 10

Losing One's Mind and Losing One's Place

A Psychosocial Model of Dementia

Chris Gilleard

The problem of mental infirmity in old age is of concern to more and more people in our present day 'ageing societies'. Conceptualisation of the problem is complex because of the multiple levels at which it can be engaged and the multiple agencies and institutions with an interest in the topic. For the pharmaceutical industry there is the challenge to produce the pills that retard or reverse intellectual decay; for the clinician there is the task of managing to keep beds free, families coping and patients independent while maintaining morale in the Cinderella services of psychogeriatrics and geriatrics; for the policy analyst and the health economist there is the question of costs, the expenses of dementia, the competition for resources and the viability and exchangeability of differing systems of care. For the theologian there is the dilemma of the naturalness of senility, the nature of suffering and the selection of an appropriate pastoral response to those suffering with dementia; and for families there is the personal struggle and grief of a difficult and disorganised loss. Finally there is the very personal issue of how one copes with the erosion of one's very own personhood.

Within all these concerns lies the debate concerning the nature and implementation of an appropriate human response to the decline of mental competence in later life. This is the main issue of my chapter: namely, how we can best understand dementia in order to frame a fair and considerate societal response. Thus one can consider dementia in relation to the present welfare debate concerning community care. In his recent report to the British government, Sir Roy Griffiths stated that:

> Publicly provided services constitute only a small part of the total care provided to people in need. Families, friends, neighbours and other local people provide the majority of care in response to needs which they are uniquely well placed to identify and respond to...and...this is as it should be (Griffiths 1988).

This last phrase states the position clearly...a just policy to help those who are disabled is one that places the onus on the family and the local community to identify, assess and respond to the problem. Such a stance links a morally valued 'human rights' perspective with one that implicitly undermines the paternalism of centralised welfare state interference. Long-term care and its accompanying burdensomeness are best kept in the community; the rights of the individual to stay in his or her own home and to be looked after for better or worse by his or her own kin are set against the 'indignity' of being placed into the welfare of the state. Such individualism is viewed as both a morally superior and an economically more efficient code of living. Taken to extremes, this view scoffs at paternalism, infantilisation and welfare mollycoddling in all its forms. As the empires of central planning fall elsewhere this social philosophy heralds a new triumph of personal freedom and individualism.

Treating adults as children: determining where they live, what they do, when they go to bed, when they rise, what they eat, helping them dress, making sure they are ready for the ambulance, minibus, or the next music and movement session – these are widely viewed as the prototypical features of totalitarian/institutional care. By contrast, community care policies assert the right of the elderly person to be recognised as an adult and treated as such, and to be given respect and dignity, which also means not being made to go to bed or to get up or to eat or to bathe or to dress.

The reality of community care is not exactly like that. Once the family or neighbours have realised that there is something wrong and something needing to be done, then responses to need are initiated. The district nurse comes in to help the old man dress while chiding him for not helping more; the warden of the housing complex points out to the visiting social worker the dangerous habits and vulnerabilities of her charges, where they hide their soiled linen and how none of the family really cares; and the home help slips in and places the tea and biscuits close at hand encouraging 'gran' to drink it all up before it goes cold while she gets on and does the washing up.

Despite such everyday practices, the principle of care with dignity in the community is retained; the goal forever reasserted that one should show respect for the individuality of the client, as if by some fiat on a half-day training course one can impose a view or attitude that flies in the face of the behavioural reality of dementia care practices. In the light of these everyday contradictions it seems desirable to look once more at the nature of dementia and particularly how it is linked to the more general issue of individual mind and collective society.

To do this, I should like to consider two models of dementia (see Table 10.1). The first is one that stresses the disease of dementia – the specification of a Pick's disease, an Alzheimer's disease or a Jakob-Creutzfeldt disease. The second model sees dementia as a stage within one person's life cycle, a variant of senility, one way of growing old. In the former case dementia is something which happens to an individual, a disease affecting one's brain, more especially a disease that affects particular regions and cell and sub-cellular systems within the brain itself. The latter stresses that dementia is something that happens to individuality itself and beyond that individuality to family and social systems within which that individual possessed and provided meaning. The former model emphasises the bits that are and are not dementia, while the latter considers the global nature of decay and loss, and the involution of the person.

Table 10.1 Two models of dementia

Neuropsychobiological	*Psychosocial*
Disease of an organ system	Disorder of a person
Co-existence of healthy and diseased systems and organs system	Global deterioration of the organism, mind and family
Mind as an endogenous epigenetic product of brain structure	Mind as a constituent of a social system
Piagettian development	Vygotskian development
A search for causality	A concern for consequence

If we call the former a neuropsychobiological model we may term the latter one a psychosocial model. The research interests of those pursuing the two models reflect their distinctiveness. In neuropsychobiological research, fragmentation of function is studied – the decay of particular neurotransmitter substances, the pattern of neuropsychological deficits and the molecular distortions of neuronal function – with the explicit aim of seeking to restore to normal functions which have gone awry, damaging and distressing the patient sufferer. Psychosocial research on the other hand examines the breakdown in personal relationships, the meanings and interpretations that carers and sufferers bring to the condition, the stresses of changing relationships brought about by dementia and the strategies employed to cope with the resulting dependency and disability. The goal of such research is to help all concerned to understand and cope with that which must be endured.

One can go further and assert that these two models differ not simply in conceptualisation and research focus, but reflect fundamentally different approaches to the study of mind. Thus the neuropsychobiological view treats mind as individually and epigenetically constituted out of its own matter (a sort of Piagettian model of mental activity) while the psychosocial model treats mind as constituted out of the interactions between people (a sort of Vygotskian view of high cortical function). Mind in the former is located within the skull; in the latter in social intercourse[1].

Without losing sight of these two models, let us now return to the issue of framing an appropriate policy and an appropriate human and societal response to the problem that is dementia. We can see that we again confront a dichotomy in the current division of social versus health care models of service. If dementia is a disease (as most of the funded research would seem to indicate) and a serious and eventually fatal disease at that, then one might feel that leaving matters up to the family and local neighbourhood to decide on an appropriate response (in the absence of nuclear magnetic resonance scanners or even a small pathology lab) would be rather ill advised. Treating mentally disabled elderly people as 'normal as possible' might seem almost 'uncaring'.

On the other hand, if dementia is just one way of growing old, an unfortunate but not infrequent way of ending one's days, then it would seem right and just that retaining one's place in the community is perhaps the best way of preserving one's mind and identity for as long as possible. The question that lies behind the concept of community care for the elderly mentally infirm is whether indeed by placing one's mind as well as one's body firmly within the community one can retain sufficient adult status to retain a mind of one's own, or whether by relinquishing it to the health service there is any real chance of it being preserved or restored.

To pursue this theme a little further afield, let us look at this concept of adulthood. It seems to me to involve the presence of three essential attributes: identity, autonomy and engagement. An adult is demonstrably a grown-up identifiable personality, someone who is deemed responsible for his or her own actions and who is best identified by the network of past and present roles and relationships that he or she has formed during the mutual interchange that is human development. Still, it is probably a mistake to define adulthood as just a place, even if it is a place in history, a place in geography and a place in society. The internal mechanisms of intelligence, our active information processing capacities, help form each adult's identity as much as others' reflected judgements. In a recent American study of street down-and-outs, the researchers clearly illustrated how even those at the bottom of the social heap strove to actively form and sustain identity and value in their communications with others (Snow and Anderson 1987). Likewise, the exercise of choice involves actively determining the possibility of alternative courses of action and not simply responding to the offer of a couple of different boxes with food inside one but not in the other. Even the establishment and maintenance of a place within the social world is not just a matter of being someone's brother or someone's wife; it requires a history both of having done things to and having done things with others and, as a result, having expectations about what one's deeds may have produced in reciprocity. In short, adulthood seems to involve agency, the exercise and not just the presence of personhood.

It is at this point that the improbability of forever retaining a place in the community for the person with dementia seems so evident. For it seems losing one's mind is also losing one's place in the adult world. But we cannot stop there. We also need to recognise that the attribution of agency, the determination of intent is a feature not of the material but of the social world. Here lies a further dilemma.

If others, the 'local' people, the friends, the families and the neighbours that Griffiths (1988) talks about, are really to be empowered to identify and respond to needs then we (the state and its agents) must listen to and accept their views. If they attribute adulthood-personhood to the elderly mentally infirm then community care would seem to be working. The state will be untroubled. But if they explicitly insist that the dementing person is not able to exercise adulthood, is in fact mentally ill and thereby incompetent, then the social care model embodied in Griffiths and most community care policy documents in this and other countries must, to be consistent, accept this appraisal. This means it must attempt to establish a more appropriate relationship than that which seeks to treat as normally as possible a human being whose personal demise should involve at the least a minimum of human suffering. The creation of thousands of miniature Nursing Homes and Hospitals throughout the country is not normal; the absence of standards of homecare is equally as worrying as the growth of an unmonitored private rest home industry. But most worrying of all is that this psychosocial view of looking after damaged, disabled or deteriorating minds is every bit as confused as the mentally infirm themselves.

Rather than replace this model with an illness model, however, we need to unravel some of this confusion. We should recognise that the exercise of adulthood is both a social and a psychological phenomenon. Active processing of, and engaging with, one's material and social environment is complemented by the interpretations and attributions of others. The over-ascription of agency by others to others is a well established phenomenon in social psychology. Where there is movement our eyes seem to tell us there is also intent. This tendency to err on the side of agency and adulthood makes most families, friends and neighbours treat the elderly mentally infirm, at least in the earlier stages, as responsible people who, when acting in harmful or potentially harmful ways, are likely to be encouraged to 'take more care'. The professional who enters this situation with the alternative explanation of illness may seek to correct these misattributions. Having done so, the same professional may proceed to re-attribute responsibility back to a system of care that has now fragmented the problem with an illness model which strategically excludes any hospital solution except when the social circumstances become intolerable.

Attributions of incompetence due to illness may successfully remove the autonomy of adult intent from the actions of the dementing person. Nevertheless, our need to attribute responsibility somehow leaves the situation unclear. Competence in the medico-legal sense, I understand, is 'decision specific' and cannot be extended to the person independently of his or her actions. Should then each action and each potential 'error' be the responsibility of a particular person at a particular time in a particular place? Should that person, that caregiver, that kinperson be informed of their responsibility? And how should one imagine that they would accept this extension of another's personhood to themselves? At some times, in some places, under some circumstances...Again the illness model fragments within its legal framework the social care it appears to prescribe.

So at present within the social care model, when a relative is treated simply as a co-carer (along with the health and social services representatives) responsibility remains equally diffuse and the sufferer's competence now accepted, now rejected according to practice and circumstance, while both neglect and uncertainty continue to characterise responses to dementia. In practice, the conceptual systems blur. At times a model of illness may be employed while at other times a model of a life cycle state of senility may prevail, and care remains in several minds.

Before we embark upon any policy-based approach to frame responses to dementia, before we assume a case management model of placing the dementing person 'in care' (albeit a social care that lacks institutional boundaries), or before we contemplate a pioneering medical dementia service that investigates and treats, but fails to care, we must seek to resolve this issue of mind and society, and the endogenous/exogenous division of personhood. If the pattern and process of inner decay, the loss of mind, is not subject to marked external influences, then the decay of this inner base of personhood is irrelevant to when and what care takes place. If on the other hand the pattern of external decay, the loss of place, and especially the attributions others make concerning the elderly individual's autonomy, identity and engagement are markedly affected by external influences, then clearly community care (which means individualised care) is preferable.

A psychosocial model of dementia cannot be predicated upon a view that argues that the inner decay of mind is socially constructed; it can however assert that the place of that mind, the external significance of that person is indeed the product of the external, social response to the person. By electing to relocate responsibility for the dementing person within a social system which explicitly accepts that responsibility, recognises the person's identity, and is engaged with that person, then that social system is unlikely to fragment its responsibility and lose the person's place in the world. In other words we can move on to consider achieving autonomy, identity and engagement for the system that cares for the person suffering with dementia. We can empower families, and we can empower institutions. More importantly we can empower the caregivers within the family system and the careworkers within the institution.

The recognition that an adult's life and personhood exist both inside and outside the individual provides an avenue by which our society can clearly think through its responsibilities for maintaining citizenship, personhood and individuality for all adults, irrespective of their individual competency. Moreover, by locating care in a social system, we do not exclude the significance of medicine in the care of persons who are ill. But the exercise of social autonomy in place of individualistic autonomy when personal competence fails means that one can no longer criticise the relative, neighbour or careworker if they fail to consult a doctor over the health of a dementing person, at least no more than if they were to fail to consult a doctor on their own account.

If the nature of the age-related changes in brain tissue should prove reparable or remediable, then there would likely be changes in the external attributions that present social systems make concerning the elderly mentally infirm person, and the social policy issues would themselves fade away or be replaced by other issues. In any psychosocial model of dementia there is an historical dynamic that creates anticipated life courses, and these are themselves subject to social developmental change. What we think of our fellow dementing citizens is a part of, and a place in, our collective consciousnesses and that place itself is a function of the institutions and practices we create in response to our various perceptions of the problem. How much, by clarifying our perceptions of the problem, we can really achieve a better (more autonomous, more identifiable, and more engaged) place for dementing people remains to be seen. Improving the autonomy of care systems is one avenue for action oriented research, but there is a need for continuing thought and greater consideration of these issues between carers and gerontologists. In the end I believe that this debate can best progress when it is, as I have tried to show, located within the existing dialogue between the psychological and sociological explanations of human development.

For mind, in the psychosocial model, is made manifest by the structure and dynamic of social forces; it represents both a particular internal system and a point in a network of such systems. Dementia represents a decay from within a particular system but it is also a loss from that network of information systems which gives a place to a person. The memory of that person, the ego as personal historian (Greenwald 1982), is sustained by other minds to an increasing degree as dementia increases in severity. It is fitting therefore that this collective ego increasingly replaces the personal ego as an agent for decision making and as a source for engaging the person in an appropriate social time and place. This process is of course a dynamic one, and subject to continuous negotiation. The issue of attributing and re-attributing responsibility is never fixed, but the direction it moves in is – and that is away from the individual and toward the collective. In societies where responsibility is inherently perceived to lie with the collective throughout adult life (relatively speaking of course) one suspects that the dilemma posed by dementia is both less acute and less significant. In our own societies, where adulthood and independence of mind are so intimately linked, the problem of dementia is consequently a severe one. Even so, it is not an all or none affair and we must learn to live without precise mental boundaries if we are to do justice to our experience of dementia.

Notes

1. The contrast between Piagettian and Vygotskian views of mental development is that of a timeless, universalistic biologically driven stage theory of mental growth (Piaget) versus that of an historically determinate, social relational view of mental growth (Vygotsky).

   Thus Vygotsky states:

   > There is not the slightest bit of hope of finding the origins of purposeful action in the height of the intellect or in the depths of the brain...to find the origins of purposeful action one must transcend the limitations of the organism. The source of human consciousness...should...be sought...in the social history of mankind (cited in Van der Veer and Ijzendoorn 1985. For a detailed account, see Vygotsky 1978)

   Piaget's views are a mix of biology and logic which he has labelled genetic epistemology. Forms of knowledge emerge through a stage like process of growth and adaptation and are already completed by the time the organism reaches biological maturity. Thus he states: 'cognitive functions constitute a specialised organ for regulating exchanges with the external world, although the instruments by which they do so are drawn from the general forms of living organisation' Piaget 1971 p.361. A succinct account of Piaget's model is given in Piaget 1970.

References

Greenwald, A. (1982) 'The totalitarian ego: fabrication and revision of personal history.' *American Psychologist* 35, 603–618.

Griffiths, Sir Roy. (1988) *Community Care: Agenda for Action.* London: HMSO.

Piaget, J. (1972) *Biology and Knowledge.* Chicago: University of Chicago Press.

Piaget, J. (1970) 'Piaget's Theory'. In Mussen, P.H. (ed) *Carmichael's Manual of Child Psychology (3(1))*. New York: Wiley and Sons Ltd. 703–732.

Snow, D.A. and Anderson, L. (1987) 'Identity work among the homeless – the verbal construction and avowal of personal identities'. *American Journal of Sociology* 92, 1336–1371.

Van der Veer, R. and Ijzendoorn, M.H. (1985) 'Vygotsky's theory of the higher psychological processes: some criticisms'. *Human Development* 28, 1–9,.

Vygotsky, L.S. (1978) *Mind and Society: the Development of Higher Psychological Processes.* Cambridge: Harvard University Press.

CHAPTER 11

Measuring the Nutritional Status of Old People

Anthea B. Lehmann

In the world of allopathic medicine most concern with undernutrition has related to people suffering because they live in an area where there is insufficient food. The second largest area of nutrition work has related to young patients in food-rich countries who have unmet increased nutritional requirements because of trauma, sepsis, or in other situations where 'auto-cannibalism' of the body occurs (a phenomenon recognised since the 1930s (Cuthbertson 1932) and which has led to the large growth in the science of supplementary tube feeding).

There appears, however, to have been a relative delay in the study of undernutrition in old age. The study of old age medicine itself is relatively new and, if only for numerical reasons, nutritionists have logically concentrated efforts on the first area of concern: that of large scale undernutrition in poor countries. In food-rich countries nutritional indices have been principally applied in relation to obesity not thinness. Nevertheless, as we attempt to disentangle the various influences on nutritional status in old people in food-rich countries, some factors contributing to the reasons for the delay in our understanding will become apparent. For example, after exhorting geriatric nutritionists to move from defense to bravery in research, Goodwin (1989) explained that 'elderly individuals have a background of symptomatology that will obscure the relatively subtle signs of a classical nutritional deficiency'.

The present challenge is to identify clearly the distinctive features of nutrition issues of old age. Pending further data, troubling questions remain: for example, is it ageist to assume that undernutrition in old people is exclusively the result of biological ageing? Or is it more ageist to attribute dangerous thinness in old people to their co-existing physical disability or low incomes? Realism is likely to be based on understanding a complex admixture of all the various influences. In this chapter I shall discuss, from a geriatrician's point of view, data which highlight certain risk factors for dangerous undernutrition in old age in food-rich countries. Normative data for possible use in assessing the nutritional status of old people in Britain are also included for reference. In addition, an example methodology for the collection of normative data will be presented, and aspects of anthropometry in relation to old people discussed.

Undernutrition in Old Age – More Dangerous Than Obesity

While in middle age and during the first two years after retirement body mass, in particular fat, may increase (Friedlander *et al* 1977, Patrick, Bassey and Fentem 1982, Rowe 1982), the subsequent trend is for a fall in body weight (Novak 1972, Burr, Millbank and Gibbs 1982, Patrick, Bassey and Fentem 1982, Steen 1988, Lehmann *et al* 1990). Undernutrition accounts for a significant morbidity and mortality in old people in food-rich countries. The contrast between the significance of obesity in young and old adults here is striking. Being underweight is numerically and prognostically of far greater importance than obesity in most groups of old people studied. Obesity was not related to heart disease in people aged over 75 years in the Framingham study (Castelli *et al* 1981) and in a study in Missouri obesity was not associated with diabetes in subjects over 69 years of age (Kohns and Tobben 1982). And, in another study, being moderately overweight was not associated with a higher mortality in old age (Andres 1980). This absence of associations may reflect, in part, the selective earlier mortality of obese subjects. Nevertheless longitudinal studies in old age do warn of the dangers of thinness – lower body weight carries a higher mortality whether measured initially in old people living at home (Mattila, Haavisto and Rajala 1986, Campbell *et al* 1990) or in patients on admission to a hospital ward (Bienia *et al* 1982; Friedman, Cambell and Caradoc-Davies 1985). The correlation between poor nutrition and the risk of hip fracture is now apparent from studies of both cross-sectional (Older, Delyth and Dickerson 1980, Bastow, Rawlings and Allison 1983, Delmi *et al* 1990) and longitudinal (Kiel *et al* 1987; Farmer *et al* 1989) design.

Immunodeficiency

Undernutrition has long been an accepted cause of immunodeficiency, and in a prospective study of fit old volunteers in New Mexico, Wayne *et al* (1990) found cell-mediated immunity (CMI) to be a powerful predictor of subsequent morbidity and mortality in people over 60 years of age. Improvement in lymphopaenia (a reduction in numbers of circulating lymphocytes) is used to monitor recovery from undernutrition, and impaired delayed-type hypersensitivity (which reflects CMI) is a recognised diagnostic test for undernutrition. Work in this area increasingly includes old people and has been reviewed by Chandra (1985, 1989). All too often pneumonia is diagnosed and treated in a thin old patient whose undernutrition has not been evaluated. Clues as to the mechanism and possible prevention of infection due to malnutrition are beginning to emerge. Undernourished old people in one study demonstrated a reduction in T cell numbers, the lymphocyte response to phytohaemagglutinin (PHA) and impaired CMI. Nutritional advice to increase their energy intake by 500 Kcal/day and provide recommended allowances for vitamins and trace elements led to improvements, after nine weeks, in CMI, T-lymphocyte number including CD4+ subset and lymphocyte proliferation in response to PHA (Chandra 1989). Zinc supplementation in moderate but not excessive dose has also been associated with significant improvements in CMI and immunoglobin response in old people (Chandra 1989).

Recent work suggests that glutamine, the most abundant non-essential amino acid in plasma and the free amino acid pool (Bergstrom *et al* 1974) may have a role in perpetuating the vicious circle of infection and undernutrition in old people (Lehmann 1991). Bulus *et al* (1989) have summarised evidence that muscle is the main source of glutamine (although in certain conditions such as acidosis the liver also becomes a net releaser of glutamine (Bulus *et al* 1989)). The large muscle pool of glutamine is rapidly depleted in response to stresses such as surgery, sepsis, starvation, diabetes, and stresses associated with raised glucocorticoids (Jepson *et al* 1988). Removal of glutamine from muscle and from plasma by splanchnic organs is faster than release and results in a fall in plasma glutamine during stress, sepsis and starvation; on recovery it is the last free amino acid in muscle to be restored to normal concentrations.

Not only does glutamine act as a labile store of nitrogen but its concentration in muscle correlates uniquely with rates of protein synthesis, thus raising the probability that it has an important regulatory role and that its repletion might be therapeutic (Millward, Jepson, and Omer 1989). Glutamine is also an important fuel source for enterocytes, has a trophic effect on intestinal mucosa (Bulus *et al* 1989), and is important for the maintenance of the intestinal mucosal barrier against endotoxins and bacteria (Bulus *et al* 1989, Burke *et al* 1989). Two groups have shown that lymphocyte function requires an adequate concentration of glutamine in the plasma (Newsholme, Crabtree, and Ardawi 1985, Brand *et al* 1989). It can be seen that the amino acid glutamine may have a key role linking nutrition, protein synthesis, the immune response and gut absorption whether in response to infection, starvation, illness, or trauma. In Chandra's words: 'it is attractive to postulate that nutritional engineering may alter immunocompetence and thereby reduce the burden of illness in the elderly' (Chandra 1989).

Cardiovascular Events and Hip Fractures in Winter

The yearly winter excess mortality of 40,000 old Britons may be a manifestation of the host susceptibility to the environment because of undernutrition (Keatinge 1986). The large excess mortality of old people during the winter months is attributed to cardiovascular diseases, in particular stroke and myocardial infarction, which exhibit rises in incidence that follow dips in ambient temperature with specific delays (Bull and Morton 1978). Keatinge (1986) has described the relationship between thinness and cardiovascular susceptibility to cold environment and the evidence that altered platelet function is the mechanism.

Thinness in old age predisposes the person to having a lower body core temperature when the ambient temperature drops. Fat probably has a role as an insulator (Wyndham *et al* 1968, Keatinge 1986). In addition, studies of undernutrition in children and young adults have demonstrated that an increased risk of hypothermia may be due to a failure to raise the metabolic rate in response to a cold environment – a defect which in undernourished Jamaican infants is corrected after six weeks' refeeding (Brenton, Brown and Wharton 1967, Brooke, Harris and Salvosa 1973, Smith *et al* 1983). Studies of old subjects have shown that old survivors of hypothermia have defects of heat production, shivering and peripheral vasoconstriction (Macmillan *et al* 1967); these defects were found even in healthy old people in another study (Collins *et al* 1977).

Recent work confirms that women in England with fractured hips during winter months are unusually thin compared with healthy or even medical ward age-matched groups (Mansell *et al* 1990); a prospective study of 3600 old white women in the USA similarly related low body mass index and arm anthropometry to a doubling of risk of hip fracture over the subsequent 10 years (Farmer *et al* 1989). Old white women who sustain hip fractures are, as a group, disproportionately thin. Obesity protects, to some extent, against osteoporosis.

In order to investigate further the relationship between cold susceptibility and undernutrition in hip fracture survivors, Fellows *et al* (1985) measured the rise in metabolic rate in response to cold in eight normally nourished and six undernourished women recovering from fractured femur, and this thermo-regulatory response was significantly impaired in the undernourished group. These are similar to the findings in undernourished children. In an earlier study it was found that undernourished women sustaining hip fractures in winter had lower body temperatures and were likely to fall indoors while the well-nourished sustained fractures out-of-doors (Bastow, Rawlings and Allison 1983). These results may be related to mental disturbance and ataxia both of which have previously been reported to result from hypothermia (Keatinge 1986, Golden 1973). Thus undernutrition predisposes to hypothermia that may be subacute. The result may be hip fracture, hypothermia, or acute cardiovascular events; the incidence of all these increases markedly in the UK in winter.

Many Other Consequences of Undernutrition

To this list the well-known consequences of undernutrition such as pressure sores (Pinchcofsky-Devin and Kaminski 1986, Breslow *et al* 1987) and infections (Chandra 1989) so often seen in old patients, and in whom the diagnosis of undernutrition may be missed, can be added with all the well described syndromes of specific nutrient deficiencies.

Prevalence of Undernutrition in Old Age

Prevalence data for old people commonly prompt two questions. First, is the undernutrition purely the consequence of other advanced illness, e.g. cancer or dementia, or is it a medical problem warranting separate management strategies? And second, how is a case defined? Indeed, if these questions are not specifically addressed, pure prevalence data are either meaningless or specific to only tightly defined populations of old people. The increasing prevalence of multiple pathology with age naturally explains the difficulties both in the definition of what is normative, and deciding whether to categorise, for example, well cared for but thin dying patients as undernourished.

One of the most quoted prevalence studies is that reported in Britain by the Department of Health and Social Security (DHSS) in 1979. The different interpretations of its results highlight the difficulties of geriatric nutrition. Out of a sample of 365 people aged over 65 the report records that 26 (7%) were diagnosed as clinically malnourished (clinical and biochemical diagnosis). All but one of these was said to be undernourished because of co-existing disease (e.g. bronchitis, dementia). It has been argued that this study showed that undernutrition is rarely a problem in its own right and that the other conditions were the primary problem. Others have argued that undernutrition is associated with many common diseases in old age, and therefore a lot of people are at risk. The DHSS study also demonstrated that being housebound, low income, and for men, living alone, were (less publicised) factors also correlated with poor nutritional status. In contrast to this study, physical illness per se did not account for the undernutrition of old people living in the community in a large recent study in northern Italy (Bianchetti *et al* 1990), but rather impaired functional status was among the important correlates.

Community studies have rarely defined the numbers of subjects in whom undernutrition was exclusively the primary problem. The range of figures obtained in community studies for prevalence of undernutrition in old age (see Lehmann 1989) is extremely wide (2–82%). The range is explained, at least in part, by the different methods of case definition (e.g. dietary, biochemical, clinical and anthropometric) and may also reflect sampling and population differences. There is one hospital study, albeit on a specialised ward, in which an attempt was made to define numbers of people in whom undernutrition was a primary rather than a secondary health problem; McEvoy, Dutton and James (1983) report that 31 out of 55 thin patients on this ward were thin because of poor diet.

Ethical issues contribute to the difficulties of case definition, and cultural contexts differ on either side of the Atlantic. In the USA concern is expressed regarding the 'epidemic of undernutrition in nursing homes' which is attributed to 'ignorance and the lack of adequate funds being spent on feeding the institutionalised elderly' (Morley 1989). In the UK this population (who may or may not be comparable) include a majority of people perceived as a severely disabled group, and general practitioners and geriatricians would rarely consider long-term tube feeding in patients permanently so disabled. As a consequence they are rarely given the label malnourished which would imply the need to 'treat'. Morley (1989) states that physicians frequently misjudge the patient's perception of quality of life and a recent study of cancer patients (mean age 60 years) supports this (Slevin *et al* 1990), thus reinforcing the conclusion that the manner in which these difficult decisions are made regarding treatment, and therefore case definition, clearly needs to involve patients where possible. Rudman and Feller (1989) have highlighted the variation and case mix of nursing home residents, but with the increased use of private nursing home places in the UK (where geriatricians are excluded unless specifically invited by the general practitioners), there is now a growing number of disparate old people we know surprisingly little about as a group. Thus, differing case definitions account for descriptions that range from old people requiring nursing care as suffering from an epidemic of starvation in the USA (Rudman and Feller 1989) to low values for anthropometry and vitamin levels being seen as 'indicators of inanition...in patients with poor appetite,...malignancy and...in hospitalised elderly' (Kemm and Allcock 1984) in the UK.

Factors Associated with Undernutrition

While the variety of methodologies and community studies have failed to produce a unanimous quantifiable prevalence figure, these studies have highlighted which groups of old people may benefit from special attention to their nutrition. The co-existing diagnoses associated with thinness in old age are listed in Table 11.1 (Goodwin 1989). The roles of reduced dietary intake and increased demand in these particular groups have been reviewed (Lehmann 1989). Recently, research has focused on some of the causal mechanisms (e.g. the cachexia of heart failure may be mediated by tumour necrosis factor (Levine *et al* 1990)). Studies of the relationships between both income and mobility and the nutritional health of old people are reviewed below.

Low Income

The literature regarding socio-economic factors correlated with undernutrition of old people in food-rich countries (i.e. the possible causes of 'starvation in the midst of plenty') has already been reviewed (Lehmann 1989). Data collected using a range of methodologies have demonstrated the overriding effect of poverty on diet in the old age group. Low income exceeded the effects of living arrangements (Ryan and Bower 1989) or age within the older group (Kohrs, Czajka-Narins and Nordstrom 1989). A community study sample representative of the north Italian old population included 1303

Table 11.1 Factors affecting nutritional status in elderly people

Medical Health Status
Chronic illness
Acute illness
Oral/dental health status
Depression
Social support/isolation
Level of activity
Institutionalization
Cognitive status
Medication
Economic status
Ethnic status
Effect of prescribed, therapeutic diets
Other factors limiting food choice (meal sites, etc)
Effect of major life events

Source: Reproduced with kind permission of J.S. Goodwin and the American Society of Clinical Nutrition.

people aged 70–75 years and used 24 hour dietary recall (Bianchetti *et al* 1990). Being on a low income was associated with significantly higher proportions on inadequate intakes of protein (17%), vitamin B12 (36%), vitamin A (44%), and iron (33%) in men; and B12 (38%), iron (38%) and niacin (28%) in women. (This study showed functional status and affective status to be associated with a higher prevalence of inadequate diet, but physical health status per se was not. It is, however, unfortunate that multivariate techniques for independent correlations were not used in this study). Economic and educational factors correlated with nutritional intake but rurality did not in the sample of 4000 Americans aged 60–74 years in the first National Health and Nutrition Survey (NHANES) study (Norton and Wozny 1984). In another study from the USA among old men living alone, low income was a predictor of undernutrition (Garry *et al* 1982).

The absence of such data in the UK is striking, although the ethics of investigating what might now seem obvious could be questioned. In 1967 Brockington and Lempert had already demonstrated that old people who were able to supplement their income had a better diet than those entirely dependent on a retirement pension. Members of the British Dietetic Association have recently expressed concern that their experience suggests income is inadequate for the nutritional needs of children, the elderly, pregnant women, ethnic minorities, mentally ill, and mentally handicapped people in Britain (Hanes and de Looy 1987). Low income directly or indirectly (Wicks 1978, Collins 1987) contributes to the lack of adequate heating and, as discussed above, the effect of this is compounded by undernutrition.

Reduced Mobility

Physical disability correlates closely in old age with undernutrition – as defined using dietary intake, anthropometric or metabolic balance measurements (Morgan *et al* 1986, Bunker *et al* 1987). In the absence of acute trauma or inflammation, energy intake should, and usually does, vary with energy expenditure (Bunker *et al* 1987, James, Ralph and Ferro-Luzzi 1989). However, whether such subjects should be advised to increase or decrease their protein intakes is, surprisingly, still unclear. Two early studies demonstrated negative nitrogen balance developing in fit young volunteers experimentally immobilized in plaster (Deitrick, Whedon and Shorr 1948, Schonheyder, Heilskov and Olesen 1954). In the study of Schonheyder *et al*, this occurred despite a protein intake of 1.25 g/kg/day and it was thought that the negative nitrogen balance was due to reduced protein synthesis. A more recent study on young volunteers suggests that during the first week of experimental immobilization a reduction in protein synthesis can occur which is, however, avoided if protein intake is maintained at 1 g/kg/day instead of 0.6 g/kg/day; no change in protein breakdown was recorded (Stuart *et al* 1990).

In contrast, studies using comparable leucine turnover methodology on old people in whom long-term reduced mobility was the only problem likely to influence protein turnover (and in whom nutrition was adequate), protein synthesis and breakdown were significantly faster than in their age-matched ambulant peers. Although the mean protein balance remained positive and similar to that of the ambulant control group, it might be more precarious and variance was much higher than in the control group (Norton and Wozny 1984). Young fit volunteers on complete bed rest for six days may not be comparable with old people in a stable state whose physical disability has been present for more than six weeks. Recent work on the cortisol rise during immobility in old age has suggested that this is stress not mobility-related (Roberts *et al* 1990). Stress may, therefore, account for the increased protein breakdown observed in old immobile patients (Lehmann *et al* 1989, Roberts *et al* 1990). In some of these old people who are immobile and stressed, therefore, muscle weakness may be the adult equivalent of the stunted growth observed in emotionally deprived children, a well-recognised manifestation of impaired protein balance resulting from psychological stress (Sinclair 1989, Donnet *et al* 1982).

Protein utilisation, certainly in young adults, is more efficient if energy intake is more than adequate (Kishi, Miyatani and Inove 1978), but this may be jeopardized in old age by poverty or disability. In addition, the energy expenditure when carrying out given tasks – even resting in bed, or sitting, standing, walking, or cooking – is greater in old people than in young, but the time spent carrying out such tasks may be reduced in certain individuals (James *et al* 1989). Whether protein requirements in old age during immobility are greater or smaller than in ambulant subjects remains controversial.

Measuring Nutritional Status – Anthropometry

Anthropometry refers to non-invasive measurement of body size and may include indirect measures of the amounts of fat and muscle in the body. The difficulties of anthropometry in older age groups have been a main source of delay in our understanding of nutrition issues in old age. There are three main difficulties. First, the significance of an abnormal result in old age is complex since the variance of most measurements increases with age and multiple pathology is increasingly common. Second, the difficulty in defining appropriate populations from whom to derive normative data have been considerable. Finally, there are considerable technical and conceptual difficulties making measures such as height or peripheral fat less useful. (The reliability of these indices decreases while the variance increases in old age, and they become less representative of e.g. skeletal size and total body fat respectively).

Anthropometry, the science of measuring body size and composition, is still very much in evolution in relation to old people. In a population with increasingly frequent multiple pathology, a low body measurement (e.g. weight for height) correlates less closely with the diagnosis of under-nutrition, primary or secondary, than in a young or young adult population. Increasingly, a diagnosis of undernutrition requires a medical history, clinical examination and sometimes investigations. When anorexia and weight loss co-exist, investigations are usually required to eludicate the primary cause of this vicious circle. Anorexia (Allison 1986) or intestinal microbial overgrowth (Gracey 1981) may be consequences of undernutrition; indeed, intestinal microbial overgrowth may be present in health in old people (Hellemans *et al* 1984). Clinicians cannot deduce a diagnosis of inadequate diet by anthropometric measurements quite as directly in old patients as in most younger patients.

It is clear that normative anthropometric data should be derived from representative samples of mobile healthy old people of comparable genetic constitution (Benn 1971, Lehmann *et al* 1990). Social class also must be defined when collecting or using normative anthropometric data since it affects adult height attained (Donnet *et al* 1982, Tanner 1989) and therefore needs to be comparable in the control and target populations. Some authors have dismissed healthy volunteers as non-representative, an 'elite' (Kemm and Allcock 1984). Anthropometry, par excellence, exemplifies the dilemmas in geriatric research of defining and measuring normal values. This point has been made by Rowe and Khan (1987) discussing the limitations of the 'gerontology of the usual' and by Rosenburg (1989) describing the 'normative versus the normal'. The centripetal re-distribution of fat (Clemente *et al* 1973, Mitchell and Lipschitz 1982, Steen 1988) and loss of height (Trotter and Gleser 1951, Dequeker, Baeyens and Claessens 1969) that occur during ageing are variable, and demonstrate well the widening variance of many measurements during ageing; their reliability as indices of body composition is reduced significantly in old age.

Measuring Skeletal Size – Using Limb Length Rather Than Height

The curvature of the spine and the inability to stand, of many patients whose body composition one would like to measure limit the use of height measurements if only for technical reasons. Although spinal changes account for most height loss (Trotter and Gleser 1951), lower limb contractures, or bowing, may also contribute (Kuczmarski 1989). Loss of height in old age is mainly loss of sitting height (Chumlea *et al* 1988), and is attributed to disc space loss, osteoporotic vertebral collapses and kyphosis. In a longitudinal study of white, healthy, middle class men and women in the USA aged 60–80 years, the rate of decrease in height was 0.5 cm/year (Arnetz *et al* 1983). In an older group living in sheltered flats in Sweden, average height loss over six months was of 1.4 cm (Haboubi 1990); in a comparable experimental group height loss was totally prevented ($p<0.01$) by introduction of a social activation programme (Haboubi 1990). Height is therefore not only awkward, it is an almost fluid index of skeletal size in old age.

New methods for measurement of skeletal size are mainly long bone measurements or calculations based on these (Florey 1970, Chumlea *et al* 1985, Bassey 1986, Dallosso *et al* 1986, Kwok and Whitelaw 1989, Piette *et al* 1990). It seems most straightforward, however, to deal with actual measurements (e.g. span or demi-span rather than notional calculations of possible previous body height.

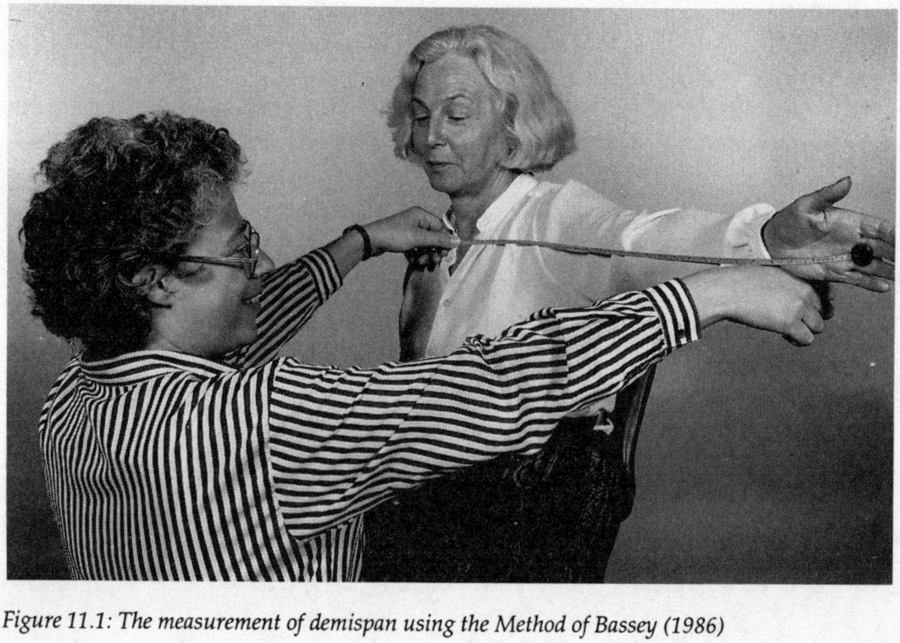

Figure 11.1: The measurement of demispan using the Method of Bassey (1986)

We have recently reported normative data based on a community study using half total arm span or demi-span (Lehmann *et al* 1990). Demi-span (DS) was already known to correlate with height in younger adults (Florey 1970); its measurement is easily learnt and carried out by one observer (see Figure 11.1). The coefficient of variation on retest and between observers was less than 1%. The methodology is convenient for collection of normative data since no undressing is required, and in the clinical setting where people often cannot stand unaided, measurements can be carried out sitting or lying. Posture appears not to influence the measurement (Lehmann *et al* 1990). Participants in this study were randomly drawn from a sample of old people living in the community. The data were collected as part of the first stage of the Nottingham Longitudinal Study of Activity and Ageing (NLSAA: see below). Only respondents able to stand without help contributed to data in Table 11.2.

Table 11.2 Deciles for weight for skeletal size, weight, and demi-span.

	Women					
	65–74 years			*75 + years*		
percentile	*mindex (kg/m)*	*weight (kg)*	*demi-span (cm)*	*mindex (kg/m)*	*weight (kg)*	*demi-span (cm)*
10	68.3	50	69.6	63.1	45	68.0
20	73.3	54	71.0	68.4	49	70.0
30	77.8	57	72.2	73.6	52	71.1
40	82.2	60	72.8	78.1	56	71.9
50	84.8	63	73.6	81.7	59	72.5
60	88.4	66	74.5	85.3	62	73.5
70	92.3	69	75.4	88.4	66	74.3
80	99.9	74	76.8	94.6	69	75.5
90	110.6	83	78.6	102.2	74	77.1
	Men					
	65–74 years			*75 + years*		
percentile	*demiquet (kg/m2)*			*demiquet (kg/m2)*		
10	87.6	57	76.8	84.5	53	75.4
20	96.1	62	78.3	92.8	57	77.0
30	99.6	65	79.5	98.9	62	77.8
40	102.4	68	80.1	103.1	66	79.0
50	106.7	71	81.4	106.3	69	80.0
60	111.6	75	82.5	109.1	72	81.3
70	117.1	79	83.8	113.4	76	82.9
80	123.7	84	85.0	119.3	78	83.8
90	130.7	89	86.9	125.0	84	85.5

Source: From Lehmann *et al* (1989). Printed with kind permission of Churchill Livingstone, Edinburgh.

Note: Demiquet is weight (kg) divided by demi-span (m) squared and mindex is weight (kg) divided by demi-span (m)

Body Mass Indices

Given a convenient measure of skeletal size, body weight measurements that are expressed in relation to skeletal size, can be used as an index of fatness or thinness. The most useful such index is one that is independent of skeletal size itself (Benn 1971, Lee, Kolonel and Hinds 1981, Constans *et al* 1990). The optimal exact ratio that has these characteristics (e.g. whether weight divided by skeletal size, or weight divided by skeletal size squared) depends on the shapes and sizes of subjects: their height, width and depth so to speak. Not surprisingly, different genetic groups, as well as the gender groups, may need a different ratio (Benn 1971, Lee *et al* 1981, Constans *et al* 1990) of weight / skeletal size (in terms of the power of the denominator) to produce a ratio itself independent of skeletal size. Florey (1970) reported that in the Framingham study while weight / height2 (Goodwin 1989) was the best ratio for white males (taking the whole adult age range as one group), weight / height was the best ratio for women. Similar results were obtained in old people in the Nottingham study (Lehmann *et al* 1990). Norms for these indices are in Table 11.2. (We have called weight / demi-span2 the 'demiquet' analagous to the Quetelet index, and weight / demi-span the 'mindex', i.e. mass index).

Table 11.3 The close correlation between total body weight and weight–corrected–for–skeletal–size in old people

	Pearson Correlation Coefficient	*p (2–tailed)*
Men		
Correlating weight with demiquet i.e. weight / demi-span2		
65–74 age group	0.81	<0.001
75 + age group	0.79	<0.001
Women		
Correlating weight with mindex i.e. weight / demi-span		
65–74 age group	0.97	<0.001
75 + age group	0.97	<0.001

Source: (Data from the Nottingham Longitudinal Study of Activity and Ageing)

It should be re-iterated that this sort of data is urgently needed for age-ranges throughout populations (Blackburn and Thornton 1979, Heymsfield *et al* 1982), and that new cohorts are likely to need new norms (Rowe 1982). In addition to these anthropometric norms, we also found that in old people in Nottingham total weight correlated very closely with weight-corrected-for-skeletal-size [see Table 11.3]. It can probably be assumed, therefore, that except for very tall or very short subjects, body weight itself is very useful in absolute terms. For most studies, however, exclusion of tall or short subjects would produce an awkward protocol.

Measuring the Body Compartments: Problems of Skinfold Measurements

For routine anthropometric uses the simple theoretical division of the body into fat and non-fat has been used, calculated typically from measures of skinfold thickness. For example, for bedside measurement of fatty tissue, triceps skinfold thickness can be carried out, and with a variety of equations using measures of arm circumference the 'lean' tissue can be quantified as arm muscle circumference or arm muscle area, the latter being considered more representative (Chumlea *et al* 1989). The equations and techniques continue to be modified and extensively reviewed (Friedlander *et al* 1977, Frost and Corish 1989). The errors resulting from skinfold thickness measurements are notorious, and are increased in older subjects (Heymsfield *et al* 1989, Sullivan *et al* 1989, Rudman *et al* 1990). Of all simple physical anthropometric measures of US veterans (e.g. arm circumference, abdominal girth, limb lengths) Friedlander *et al* (1977) reported skinfolds to have the lowest reliability. The technical difficulties appear to be improved by repeated training but in some old subjects a slight difference (of only 1cm) in the site of skinfold measurement can produce readings differing by 80–144% (Rudman *et al* 1990). The subcutaneous fat of old people (especially over the triceps) may, presumably, be unevenly distributed and its compressibility also contributes to huge variances. Sullivan *et al* (1989) have shown that the error of triceps skinfold measurements increases with the value of that measurement. Frost and Cornish (1989) obtained this same relationship of error increasing with body mass in their study carried out by trained dietitians.

During ageing the trend is for a reduction in lean body mass and an increase in total body fat (Novak 1972; Steen 1988; Chumlea and Baumgartner 1989) although exercise (Patrick, Bassey and Fenlem 1982) or even growth hormone (Deurenberg *et al* 1990) may over-ride these trends. At the same time fat undergoes a variable centripetal redistribution towards the trunk (Deurenberg *et al* 1990) but it is also significantly redistributed internally (Lukaski 1987) such that abdominal girth or truncal skinfold measurements may also fail to be representative of total body fat. As Heymsfield *et al* (1989) state: 'in a context of the changing composition of body compartments during ageing, the advent of new methodologies that are not 'age-sensitive' is to be welcomed'.

New Theoretical Models for Body Composition

The development of new methodologies coincides with the development of the 4-compartment model rather than the 2-compartment model, particularly since the assumptions that the composition of fat-free mass is unchanged during ageing is now deemed to be false (Lukaski 1987, Chumlea and Baumgartner 1989, Bouchard, Bray and Hubbard 1990). Although the density of fat is constant between individuals, the composition of the rest of the body, i.e. the proportions of water, protein, osseous (bony) and non-osseous minerals is not (Lukaski 1987). Clearly, if only a measure of fat were required, and this were measured directly and not by subtraction of an inaccurate index of lean body mass, then the subdivisions of the non-fat compartment are irrelevant. If only one component of the non-fat compartment is measured, or if the size of one component of this compartment is what is required, then the two-compartment model is unsatisfactory and may introduce errors of up to 15% (Lukaski 1987).

New Technologies

Researchers are at present evaluating the new methodologies to measure the various compartments. Bioelectrical impedance measures can be carried out painlessly using easily transported equipment to calculate total fat-free mass. Deurenberg *et al* (1990) have validated the equations for this in old people against the 'gold standard' or under-water weighing (e.g. hydrodensitometry). Equations derived from younger adults, however, overestimated fat by as much as 6kg in old people. The new age-specific equations are calculations of total fat-free mass derived from height, electrical resistance, body weight and thigh circumference. Other new methodologies which better quantify the four body compartments include absorptiometry, computerised tomography, neutron activation analysis, B-mode ultrasound, magnetic resonance imaging, and neutron inelastic scattering. It is only with bioelectrical impedance measurements that validation of age-specific equations has been carried out. In addition, the other technologies are, in general, too cumbersome or expensive for the clinical setting.

Nutritional Indices from the Nottingham Longitudinal Study of Activity and Ageing

The Nottingham Longitudinal Study of Activity and Ageing was set up in 1983 to assess the role of life style and Customary Physical Activity (CPA) in promoting and maintaining health and psychological well-being in later life. The first population survey was conducted between May and September 1985, during which time 1042 people randomly sampled from the community, and demographically representative of the British elderly population, were interviewed in their own homes. The interview questionnaire contained a total of 318 items and covered aspects of health, life style, demographic and socio-economic status, and was followed by selected anthropometric measurements.

Of those successfully interviewed in the first wave (1985) data collection for the NLSAA, 14 were unable to co-operate with the anthropometric measurements, 68 could not stand unaided on the scales, and 28 were lost for miscellaneous reasons. The success rate for complete measurements on both demi-span and weight (n = 890) was 90%.

Reported Health and Well-being

The questionnaire elicited information about a wide range of health problems, social class and customary physical acitivity. A profile of psychological well-being included the Life Satisfaction Index, assessments of anxiety, depression, and Social Engagement scale, and duration of time since the loss of a partner. Physical health was assessed on a 14-point health index, incorporating perceived health, prescribed drugs, and the presence of a variety of symptoms (see Morgan *et al*, 1987, Dalloso *et al*, 1988).

Body mass was measured in respondents without shoes, lightly clothed, standing on bathroom scales. The scales were calibrated initially and checked regularly against Roman arm scales by duplicate weighing of at least two individuals of different sizes. They were precise and accurate to ±0.5 kg and read to 130 kg. Shoulder flexibility was measured according to the method previously described as an index of the range of arm abduction, (see Bassey *et al*, 1989).

Hand-grip strength was measured in standard posture using a strain-gauged dynamometer (best score from either hand). The dynamometer, which was custom-built, was not sensitive to the position of force application and had a peak hold display (Bassey, Dudley and Harries 1986).

Analysis

Men and women were treated separately throughout. Data are reported as mean values with 2-tailed significance testing unless otherwise stated. Associations were tested using Spearman's Rank Correlation (rho) for ordinal data, Pearson's Product Moment (r) for interval data or Chi-squared for nominal data, and multiple regression analysis using controlled entry of variables. The coefficient of variation on retest and between interviewers was less than 1% for both demi-span and weight. Between interviewer variation within the survey was absent for weight and less than 2% for demi-span. For the nutritional Indices (NI), the demiquet (mass / demi-span^2 kg m-2) was used for men, the mindex (mass / demi-span kg m-1) for women.

Results

Age and Sex Differences in Anthropometry

Table 11.2 shows the sex differences in demi-span (DS) and weight. DS was normally distributed while weight was positively skewed in women. Weight and DS were both lower in older groups (follow-up data will distinguish secular from ageing changes). Mean NI were lower in the older age groups, reaching statistical significance only in women (t-test, p); the older women (75+) therefore, as a group, had significantly lower weight-for-stature than younger women (65–74).

Social Factors

Occupational class (via influences in childhood) is a known determinant of adult height, but in these old subjects it was only in the 'young old' women of the 65–74 age group that DS was correlated with occupational class (rho = 0.15, p). Ease with which £200 could be obtained in an emergency was asked of respondents as an index of economic status, but this bore no relation to NI. In the older group of old men NI negatively correlated with the duration since the loss of their partner through separation or death (rho = 0.18, $p<0.01$) and it was also only in this group (men only aged 75+) that living alone was found to be associated with thinness ($p = 0.02$). The social engagement score was significantly correlated with NI in men (rho = .14, $p<0.01$). Receipt of Meals on Wheels bore no relation to NI.

Physical Health

The number of prescribed drugs, and a range of reported symptoms bore no relation to NI, nor did the 14-item health score. Smoking, use of GP services, the presence of cardiac or stomach problems, and the occurrence of falls, also bore no relation to NI. The only significant associations found were that significantly more heavy women (high NI) than expected by chance reported high blood pressure and symptoms of arthritis, the latter defined as pain at night and stiffness in the morning ($p<0.001$).

Psychological State

Those unable to co-operate because of very advanced dementia were excluded from this analysis. Depression scores were not correlated in this study with any anthropometric measures, except the (presumed) chance finding that men who were depressed had shorter armspans (not explained by social class).

Handgrip Strength

This only correlated with NI in women aged 75+ and this was a weak correlation (r = 0.18, p.01). In contrast, in all groups handgrip strength correlated very significantly with shoulder flexibility ($p<0.001$).

Conclusions from NLSAA Cross Sectional Analyses

Nutritional Status Among Mobile Old People at Home

The relationship between class and demi-span is principally of demographic and historic interest, suggesting that women, not men, who are now old show the main skeletal consequences of poverty in childhood. Whether the very old cohort of women escaped either cause of consequence, or have undergone selective ageing, cannot be deduced at this stage of the study.

Poverty has been shown to be a risk factor for undernutrition as discussed earlier, but was not apparent in this study of relatively well 'community-living' old people. Socially isolated men, however, even in this category, were substantially thinner, a finding noted in other surveys (for review see Lehmann 1989). The lack of association between thinness and physical or psychological illness is striking. Of note for research purposes in particular is that handgrip strength cannot be seen per se as an index of nutritional status. Specific measures of muscle bulk might reveal a correlation with this, but handgrip strength appears more closely related to fitness and agility.

In general, the findings of this study suggest that in the community, old people who can stand unaided (i.e. are mobile) do not as a group show the associations of thinness with the many disorders or risk factors described in studies derived from hospital attenders or more heterogeneous samples (e.g. day centre attenders).

In the Nottingham study the diagnosis of undernutrition was not specifically sought. It differs from other community surveys of nutritional indices in community-living old people in that the sample was representative, in terms of age structure, sex, and occupational class, of old people in Britain. Many risk factors previously identified for undernutrition were not associated with thinness in this sample of old people who lived at home and can stand unaided. One explanation might be that most old people at risk were in institutions already, though from personal experience, clinical work on acute geriatric assessment wards in Nottingham does not suggest this. The precise explanation cannot be deduced from this survey, but might be that mobile or non-institutionalised old people are not susceptible to the same undernutrition risks as less screened or less mobile old people. This study reinforces the divergence between hospital-identified and community-identified old people in Britain. Within the old age groups it is as if at least two quite distinct populations emerge, distinguished by vulnerability or that even more vague word, frailty.

Acknowledgements

I am most grateful to the research team and respondents of the Nottingham Longitudinal Study of Activity and Ageing for allowing and helping me to analyse these data. I am particularly grateful to Dr Joan Bassey for help with the analyses.

References

Allison, S.P. (1986) 'Some psychological and physiological aspects of enteral nutrition'. *Gut* 27 (Suppl. 1) 18–24.

Andres, R. (1980) 'Effect of obesity on total mortality'. *International Journal of Obesity* 4, 381–86.

Arnetz, B.B., Theorell, T., Levi, L., Kallner, A. and Eneroth, P. (1983)' An experimental study of social isolation of elderly people: psychoendocrine and metabolic effects'. *Psychosomatic Medicine* 45 (5) 395–406.

Bassey, E.J. (1986) 'Demi-span as a measure of skeletal size'. *Annals of Human Biology* 13 (5) 499–502.

Bassey, E.J., Dudley, B.R. and Harries, U.J. (1986) 'A new portable strain-gauged hand-grip dynamometer'. *Journal of Physiology* 373, 6P.

Bassey, E.J., Morgan, K., Dallosso, H.M. and Ebrahim, S.B.J. (1989) 'Flexibility of the shoulder joint measured as a range of abduction in a large representative sample of men and women over 65 years of age.' *European Journal of Applied Physiology* 58, 353–60.

Bastow, M.D., Rawlings, J. and Allison, S.P. (1983) 'Undernutrition, hypothermia, and injury in elderly women with fractured femur: an injury response to altered metabolism'.*Lancet* (i) 143–46.

Benn, R.Y. (1971) 'Some mathematical properties of weight-for-height indices used as a measure of adiposity'. *British Journal of Preventative and Social Medicine* 25, 42–50.

Bergstrom, J., Furst, P., Noree, L.O. *et al* (1974) 'Intracellular free amino acid concentration in human muscle tissue'. *Journal of Applied Physiology* 36, 693–96.

Bianchetti, A., Rozzini, R., Carabellese, C., Zanetti, O. and Trabacchi, M. (1990) 'Nutritional intake, socioeconomic conditions, and health status in a large elderly population'. *Journal of the American Geriatrics Society* 38, 521–6.

Bienia, R., Ratcliff, S., Barbour, G.L. and Kummer, M. (1982) 'Malnutrition in the hospitalised geriatric patient'. *Journal of the American Geriatrics Society* 30 (7) 433–36.

Blackburn, G.L. and Thornton, P.A. (1979) 'Nutritional assessment of the hospitalised patient.' *Nutr. Clin. N. Am.* 63, 1105–8.

Bouchard, C., Bray, G.A. and Hubbard, V.S. (1990) 'Basic and clinical aspects of regional fat distribution.' *American Journal of Clinical Nutrition* 52, 946–50.

Brand, K., Fekl, W., van Hitzenstern, J., Langer, K., Lupper, P. and Schoerner, C. (1989) 'Metabolism of glutamine in lymphocytes'. *Metabolism* 38 (8) Suppl. 1 (Aug) 29–33.

Brenton, D.P., Brown, R.E. and Wharton, B.A. (1967) 'Hypothermia in kwashiorkor'. *Lancet* (i) 410–13.

Breslow, R., Hallfisch, J., Moser, P.B., Maney, D., Muller, D. and Goldberg, A. (1987) 'Nursing home patients'. *Fed. Proc.* 46, 4042.

Brockington, C.F. and Lempert, D. (1967) *The social needs of the over eighties: the Stockport survey.* Manchester: Manchester University Press.

Brooke, O.G., Harris, M. and Salvosa, C.P. (1973) 'The response of malnourished babies to cold.' *Journal of Physiology* (London) 233, 75–91.

Bull, G.M., Morton, J. (1978) 'Environment temperature and death rates'. *Age and Ageing* 7 (4) 210–24.

Bulus, N., Cersosimo, E., Ghisan, F. and Abumrad, N.N. (1989) 'Psychologic importance of glutamine'. *Metabolism: Clinical and Experimental.* 38 (8) Suppl. 1, 1–5.

Bunker, V.W., Lawson, M.S., Stansfield, M.F. and Clayton, B.E. (1987) 'Nitrogen balance studies in apparently healthy elderly and those who are housebound'. *British Journal of Nutrition* 57, 211–21.

Burke, D.J., Alverdy, J.C., Aoys, E. and Moss, G.S. (1989) 'Glutamine-supplemented total parental nutrition improves gut immune function.' Archives of Surgery 124, 1396–99.

Burr, M.L., Milbank, J.E., and Gibbs, D. (1982) 'The nutritional status of the elderly'. *Age and Ageing* 11, 89–96.

Campbell, A.J., Spears, G.R.S., Brown, J.S., Busby, W.J. and Borrie, M.J. (1990) 'Anthropometric measurements as predictors of mortality in a community population aged 70 years and over'. *Age and Ageing* 19, 131–35.

Castelli, W.P., Dawbert, T.R., Gordon, R., and Kannel, W.B. (1981) 'Lipoproteins, cardiovascular disease and death: the Framingham study.' *Archives of Internal Medicine* 141, 1128–31.

Chandra, R.K. (ed) (1985) *Nutrition, immunity and illness in the elderly.* Oxford: Pergamon Press.

Chandra, R.K. (1989) 'Nutritional regulation of immunity and risk of infection in old age'. *Immunology* 67, 141–7.

Chandra, R.K. (1989) 'Nutritional regulation of immunocompetence and risk of disease'. In Horwitz, A., Macfadyen, D.M., Munro, H. *et al* (eds), *Nutrition in the Elderly*. Oxford: Oxford University Press (for World Health Organisation).

Chumlea, W.C. and Baumgartner, R.N. (1989) 'Status of anthropometry and body composition data in elderly subjects.' *American Journal of Clinical Nutrition* 50, 1158–66.

Chumlea, W.C., Garry, P.J., Hunt, W.C. and Rhyne, R.L. (1988) 'Serial changes in stature and weight in a healthy elderly population'. *Human Biology* 60, 918–25.

Chumlea, W.C., Roche, A.F. and Steinbaugh M.L. (1989) 'Anthropometric approaches to the nutritional assessment of the elderly'. In Munro, H.N., and Danford, D. (eds) *Nutrition, aging and the elderly. Human Nutrition Vol 6* (eds) Alfin-Slater and Kritchevsky. NY, London: Plenum Press.

Chumlea, W.C., Roche, A.F. and Steinbaugh, M.L. (1985) 'Estimating stature from knee height for persons 60 to 90 years of age'. *Journal of the American Geriatrics Society* 33, 116–20.

Clemente, G., Ferro-Luzzi, A., Mariani, A., Santaroni, G. and Tranquilli, G.B. (1973) 'Evaluation of analytical models based on anthropometry and age for the prediction of body fat'. *Nutr. Rep. Int.* 7, 157–68.

Collins, K., Dore, C., Exton-Smith, A.N., Fox, R.H., Macdonald, I.C. and Woodward, P.M. (1977) 'Accidental hypothermia and impaired temperature homeostasis in the elderly'. *British Medical Journal* (i) 353–56.

Collins, K.J. (1987) 'Effects of cold on old people'. *British Journal of Hospital Medicine*, December, 506–14.

Constans, T., Bacq, Y., Bertrand, P., Beaugerie, A., Babault, C., Delarue, J. and Lamisse, F. (1990) 'The American anthropometric norms are not suitable to assess the nutritional status of a French population'. *Clinical Nutrition* 9, 168–71.

Cuthbertson, D.P. (1932) 'Observations on the disturbance of metabolism produced by injury to the limbs'. *Quarterly Journal of Medicine* 1, 223–46.

Dallosso, H., Morgan, K., Ebrahim, S *et al.* (1986) 'Health and contact with medical services among the elderly in Greater Nottingham'. *East Midland Geographer* 9, 37–44.

Dallosso, H.M., Morgan, K., Bassey, E.J., Ebrahim, S.B.J., Fentem, P.H. and Arie, T. (1988) 'Levels of customary physical activity among the old and the very old living at home'. *Epidemiology and Community Health* 42 (2) 121–7.

Deitrick, J.E., Whedon, G.D. and Shorr, E. (1948) 'Effects of immobilisation upon various metabolic and physiologic functions of normal men.' American Journal of Medicine 4, 3–36.

Delmi, M., Rapin, C.H., Bengoa, J-M., Delmas, P.D., Vasey, H. and Bonjour, J-P. (1990) 'Dietary supplementation in elderly patients with fractured neck of femur'. *Lancet* 335 (i) 1013–16.

Department of Health and Social Security (1979) 'A nutrition survey of the elderly'. *Rep. Health Soc. Subj.* No 1.16 London: HMSO.

Dequeker, J.V., Baeyens, J.P. and Claessens, J. (1969) 'The significance of stature as a clinical measurement of ageing'. *Journal of the American Geriatrics Society* 17, 169–79.

Deurenberg, P., van der Kooij, K., Evers, P. and Hulshof, T. (1990) 'Assessment of body composition by bioelectrical impedance in a population aged 60 years'. *American Journal of Clinical Nutrition* 51, 3–6.

Donnet, M.L., Cole, T.J., Scott, T.M. and Stanfield, J.P. (1981–1982) 'Diet, growth and health of infants in a disadvantaged inner city environment in Glasgow'. In

Turner, Michael R. (ed) *Nutrition and Health.* Proceedings of British Nutrition Foundation Conference. Lancaster: MTP Press Ltd, 183–95.

Ebrahim, S.B.J., Dallosso, H.M., Morgan, K., Bassey, E.J., Fentem, P.H. and Arie, T. (1988) 'Causes of ill health in a random sample of old and very old people: possibilities for prevention.' *Journal of the Royal College of Physicians of London* 22, 105–7.

Enzi, G., Gasparo, M., Biondetti, P.R., Fiore, D., Sernisa, M. and Zurlo, F. (1987) 'Subcutaneous and visceral fat distribution according to sex, age and overweight, evaluated by computed tomography'. *American Journal of Clinical Nutrition* 45, 7–13.

Evans, J.G. and Prior, I.A.M. (1969) 'Indices of obesity derived from height and weight in two Polynesian populations'. *British Journal of Preventative and Social Medicine* 23, 56–9.

Farmer, M.E., Harris, T., Madans, J.H., Wallace, R.B., Cornoni-Huntley, J. and White, J.R. (1989) 'Anthropometric indicators and hip fracture. The NHANES-I epidemiologic follow-up study'. *Journal of the American Geriatrics Society* 37, 9–16.

Fellows, I.W., Macdonald, I.A., Bennett, T. and Allison, S.P. (1985) 'The effect of undernutrition on thermoregulation in the elderly.' *Clinical Science* 69, 525–32.

Florey, C. du V. (1970) 'The use and interpretation of ponderal index and other weight-height ratios in epidemiological studies'. *Journal of Chronic Diseases* 23, 93–103.

Friedlander, J.S., Costa, P.T., Bosse, R., Ellis, E., Rhoads, J.G. and Stoudt, N.W. (1977) 'Longitudinal physique changes among healthy white veterans at Boston'. *Human Biology* 49, 541–58.

Friedman, P.J., Campbell, A.J. and Caradoc-Davies, T.H. (1985) 'Prospective trial of a new diagnostic criterion for severe wasting malnutrition in the elderly.' *Age and Ageing* 14, 149–54.

Frost, G.S. and Corish, C. (1989) 'Reproducibility of upper-arm anthropometry in subjects of differing body mass'. *Journal of Human Nutrition and Dietetics* 2, 403–6.

Garry, P.J., Goodwin, J.S., Hunt, W.C., Hooper, E.M. and Leonard, A.G. (1982) 'Nutritional status in a healthy elderly population: dietary and supplemental intakes'. *American Journal of Clinical Nutrition* 36, 332–9.

Golden, F. St. C. (1973) 'Recognition and treatment of immersion hypothermia'. *Proceedings of the Royal Society of Medicine* 66, 1053–61.

Goodwin, J.S. (1989) 'Social, psychological and physical factors affecting the nutritional status of elderly subjects: separating cause and effect'. *American Journal of Clinical Nutrition* 50, 1201–9.

Goodwin, J.S. (1989) 'Summary comments.' *American Journal of Clinical Nutrition* 50, 1234–5.

Gracey, M.S. (1981) 'Nutrition, bacteria and gut'. *British Medical Bulletin* 37, 71–5.

Haboubi, N.Y., Hudson, P.R. and Pathy, M.S. (1990) 'Measurement of height in the elderly'. *Journal of the American Geriatrics Society* 38, 1008–10.

Hanes, F.A. and de Looy, A.E. (1987) 'Can I afford the diet?' *Human Nutrition: Applied Nutrition* 41A, 1–12.

Hellemans, J., Joosten, E., Ghoos, Y., Carchon, H., Vantrappen, G., Pelemans, W. and Rutgeerts, P. (1984) 'Positive 14CO2 bile acid breath test in elderly people'. *Age and Ageing* 13, 138–43.

Heymsfield, S.B., Wang, J., Lichtman, S., Kamen, Y., Kehayias, J. and Pierson, R.N. (1989) 'Body composition in elderly subjects: a critical appraisal of clinical methodology'. *American Journal of Clinical Nutrition* 50, 1167–75.

Heymsfield, S.R., McManus, C., Smith, J., Stevens, U. and Nixon, D.W. (1982) 'Anthropometric measurement of muscle mass: revised equations for calculating bone-face arm muscle area'. *American Journal of Clinical Nutrition* 36, 680–90.

James, W.P.T., Ralph, A. and Ferro-Luzzi, A. (1989) 'Energy needs of the elderly'. In Munro, H.N. and Danford, D. (eds) *Nutrition, ageing and the elderly. Human Nutrition 6*, (eds) Alfin–Slater and Kritchevsky. NY, London: Plenum Press.

Jepson, M.M., Bates, P.C., Broadbent, P., Pell, J.M. and Millward, D.J. (1988) 'Relationship between glutamine concentration and protein synthesis in rat skeletal muscle'. *American Journal of Physiology* 255 (Endocrinol. Metab. 18) E166–72.

Keatinge, W. (1986) 'The medical problems of cold weather'. *Journal of the Royal College of Physicians of London*. 29, 283–87.

Kemm, J.R, and Allcock, J. (1984) 'The distribution of supposed indicators of nutritional status in elderly patients'. *Age and Ageing* 13, 21–8.

Kiel, D.P., Felson, D.P., Anderson, J.J. *et al.* (1987) 'Hip fracture and the use of oestrogens in postmenopausal women: the Framingham study'. *New England Journal of Medicine* 317, 1169–74.

Kishi, K., Miyatani, S. and Inoue, G. (1978) 'Requirement and utilisation of egg protein by Japanese young men with marginal intakes of energy'. *Journal of Nutrition* 108, 658–69.

Kohns, M.B. and Tobben, C.K. (1982) 'Association of obesity with disease among the elderly'. *Nutr. Rep. Int.* 25, 533–41.

Kohrs, M.B., Czajka-Narins, C.M. and Nordstrom, J. (1989) 'Factors affecting nutritional status of the elderly'. In Munro, H.N., Danford, D. (eds) *Nutrition, ageing and the elderly*. London: Plenum Press.

Kuczmarski, R.J. (1989) 'Need for body composition information in elderly subjects'. *American Journal of Clinical Nutrition* 50, 1150–7.

Kwok, T. and Whitelaw, M.N. (1989) 'A new nutritional indicator. Letter to the Editor'. *Journal of the American Geriatrics Society* 37, 1100–01.

Lee, J., Kolonel, L.N. and Hinds, M.W. (1981) 'Relative merits of the weight-corrected-for-height indices'. *American Journal of Clinical Nutrition* 34, 2521–9.

Lehmann, A.B. (1989) 'Review: undernutrition in elderly people'. *Age and Ageing* 18, 339–53.

Lehmann, A.B. (1991) 'Nutrition in old age, Part II'. *Review in Old Age* (in press).

Lehmann, A.B., Bassey, E.J., Morgan, K. and Dallosso, H.M. (1990) 'Normal values for weight, skeletal size and body mass indices in 890 men and women aged over 65 years'. *Clinical Nutrition* (in press).

Lehmann, A.B., Johnston, D. and James, O.F.W. (1989) 'The effects of old age and immobility on protein turnover in human subjects with some observations on the possible role of hormones'. *Age and Ageing* 18, 148–57.

Levine, B., Kalman, J. Mayer, L., Fillit, H.M. and Packer, M. (1990) 'Elevated circulating levels of tumor necrosis factor in severe chronic heart failure'. *New England Journal of Medicine* 323 (4) 236–41.

Lukaski, H.C. (1987) 'Methods for the assessment of human body composition: traditional and new'. *American Journal of Clinical Nutrition* 46, 537–56.

Macmillan, A.L., Corbett, J.L., Johnson, R.H., Smith, A.C., Spalding, J.M.K. and Wolner, L. (1967) 'Temperature regulation in survivors of accidental hypothermia of the elderly'. *Lancet* (ii) 165–69.

Mansell, P.I., Rawlings, J., Allison, S.P., Bendall, M.J., Pearson, M., Bassey, E.J. and Bastow, M. (1990) 'Low anthropometric indices in elderly females with fractured neck of femur'. *Clinical Nutrition* 9, 190–4.

Mattila, K., Haavisto, M. and Rajala, S. (1986) 'Body mass index and mortality in the elderly'. *British Medical Journal* 292, 867–68.

McEvoy, A., Dutton, J. and James, O.F.W. (1983) 'Bacterial contamination of the small intestine is an important cause of occult malabsorption in the elderly'. *British Medical Journal* 287, 789–93.

Millward, D.J., Jepson, M.M. and Omer, A. (1989) 'Muscle glutamine concentration and protein turnover in viva malnutrition and endotoxaemia'. *Metabolism* 38 (8) Suppl. 1 (Aug) 6–13.

Mitchell, C.O. and Lipschitz, D.A. (1982) 'Arm length measurement as an alternative to height in nutritional assessment of the elderly'. *J.P.E.N.* 6 (3) 226–9.

Mitchell, C.O. and Lipschitz, D.A. (1982) 'The effects of age and sex on the routinely used measurements to assess nutritional status of hospitalised patients'. *American Journal of Clinical Nutrition* 36, 340–9.

Morgan, D.B., Newton, H.M.V., Schorah, C.J., Jewitt, M.A., Hancock, M.R. and Hullin, R.P. (1986) 'Abnormal indices of nutrition in the elderly: a study of different clinical groups'. *Age and Ageing* 15, 65–76.

Morgan, K., Dallosso, H.M., Arie, T., Byrne, E.J., Jones, R. and Waite, J. (1987) 'Mental health and psychological well-being among the old and the very old living at home'. *British Journal of Psychiatry* 150, 801–7.

Morley, J.E. (1989) 'Death by starvation. A modern American problem?'. *Journal of the American Geriatrics Assoc.* 37, 184–5.

Neugarten, B.L., Havighurst, R.J. and Tobin, S.S. (1969) 'The measurement of life satisfaction'. *Journal of Gerontology* 16, 134–43.

Newsholme, E.A., Crabtree, B. and Ardawi, M.S.M. (1985) 'Glutamine metabolism in lymphocytes: its biochemical, physiological and clinical importance'. *Quarterly Journal of Experimental Physiology* 70, 473–89.

Norton, L. and Wozny, M.C. (1984) 'Residential location and nutritional adequacy among elderly adults'. *Journal of Gerontology* 39, 592–5.

Novak, L.P. (1972) 'Aging, total body potassium, fat-free mass, and cell mass in males and females between ages 18 and 85 years'. *Journal of Gerontology* 27, 438–43.

Older, M.W.J., Delyth, E. and Dickerson, J.W.T. (1980) 'A nutrient survey in elderly women with femoral neck fracture'. *British Journal of Surgery* 67, 884–86.

Patrick, J.M., Bassey, E.J. and Fentem, P.H. (1982) 'Changes in body fat and muscle in manual workers at and after retirement'. *European Journal of Applied Physiology* 49, 187–96.

Piette, F., Querel, D., Jean, A., Favre-Berrone, M., Abalain, C., Fass, H. and Dureau, C. (1990) 'Estimation chez le sujét agé de la taille maximale atteinte au cours de la vie'. *La Révue de Gériatrie* 15 (2) 69–72.

Pinchcofsky-Devin, G.D. and Kaminski, M.V. (1986) 'Correlation of pressure sores and nutritional status'. *Journal of the American Geriatrics Society* 34, 435–40.

Roberts, N.A., Barton, R.N., Horan, M.A. and White, A. (1990) 'Adrenal function after upper femoral fracture in elderly people: persistence of stimulation and the roles of adrenocorticotrophic hormone and immobility.' *Age and Ageing* 19, 304–10.

Rosenberg, I.H. (1989) 'Summary comments'. *American Journal of Clinical Nutrition* 50, 1231–3.

Rowe, J.W. (1982) 'Research in gerontology'. In Rowe, J.W., Besdine, R.W. (eds) *Health and disease in old age*. Little, Brown and Co. (Fig 27–2 of Framingham Study data).

Rowe, J.W. and Kahn, R.L. (1987) 'Human ageing: usual and successful'. *Science 237, 143–9.*

Rudman, D. and Feller, A.G. (1989) 'Protein-calorie undernutrition in the nursing home'. *Journal of the American Geriatrics Society*. 2, 173–83.

Rudman, D., Feller, A.G., Nagraj, H.S. *et al.* (1990) 'Effects of human growth hormone in men over 60 years old'. *New England Journal of Medicine* 323, 1–6 (and 1561–3 for correspondence).

Ryan, V.C. and Bower, M.E. (1989) 'Relationship of socioeconomic status and living arrangements to nutritional intake of the older person'. *Journal of the American Dietetic Association*. 89, 1805–7.

Schonheyder, F., Heilskov, N.S.C. and Olesen, K. (1954) 'Isotopic studies on the mechanism of negative nitrogen balance produced by immobilisation'. *Scandanavian Journal of Clinical and Laboratory Investigations* 6, 178–88.

Shepherd, R.J. (1987) 'Activity patterns and nutrition in the elderly'. In *Physical activity and ageing*. London, Australia: Croom Helm.

Sinclair, D. (1989) *Factors influencing growth and maturation, in Human growth after birth*. Oxford: Oxford University Press, 150–72.

Slevin,, M.L., Stubbs, L., Plant, H.J., Wilson, P., Gregory, W.M., Armes, P.J. and Downer, S.M. (1990) 'Attitudes to chemotheraphy: comparing views of patients with cancer with those of doctors, nurses, and the general public'. *British Medical Journal* 300, 1458–60.

Smith, D.K., Ovesen, L., Chu, R., Sackel, S. and Howard, L. (1983) 'Hypothermia in a patient with anorexia nervosa'. *Metabolism* 32, 1151–54.

SSPS Inc. SPSS X (Computer System), *Users Guide, 2nd Ed.* New York: McGraw Hill.

Steen, B. (1988) 'Body composition and aging'. *Nutrition Review* 42, 45–51.

Stevenson, O. (1989) *Issues for the next decade, in Age and vulnerability: A guide to better care*. London: Edward Arnold, 100–25.

Stuart, C.A., Shangraw, R.E., Peters, E.J. and Wolfe, R.R. (1990) 'Effect of dietary protein on bed-rest-related changes in whole-body-protein synthesis'. *American Journal of Clinical Nutrition* 52, 509–14.

Sullivan, D.H., Patch, G.A., Baden, A.L. and Lipschitz, D.A. (1989) 'An approach to assessing the reliability of anthropometrics in elderly patients'. *Journal of the American Geriatrics Society* 37, 607–13.

Tanner, J.M. (1989) *The interaction of heredity and environment in the control of growth, in Foetus into man: physical growth from conception to maturity*. 2nd Edition. Ware: Castlemead Publications. 119–64.

Trotter, M. and Gleser, G. (1951) 'The effect of aging on stature'. *American Journal of Physical Anthropology* 9, 311–24.

Wayne, S.J., Rhyne, R.L., Garry, P.J. and Goodwin, J.S. (1990) 'Cell-mediated immunity as a predictor of morbidity and mortality in subjects over 60'. *Journal of Gerontology* 45 (2) M45–8.

Wicks, M. (1978) *Old and Cold*. London: Heinemann Books.

Wyndham, C.H., Williams, C.G. and Loots, H. (1968) 'Reactions to cold'. *Journal of Applied Physiology* 24, 282–87.

CHAPTER 12

Care for Elderly People at Home
The Gloucester Study

Tim Dant, Brian Gearing, Malcolm Johnson and Michael Carley

The three-year Care for Elderly People at Home (CEPH) project grew from an initiative by Gloucester Health Authority (GHA) in South West England who in 1984–5 were looking for new ways of providing community care for elderly people. The main aim of the CEPH project was to explore new ways to help elderly people who were 'at risk' remain in their own homes. An important assumption underlying the approach of the project was that for elderly people in particular, health problems are intimately tied in with social situations and that needs could not simply be categorized as 'social' or 'medical'. Thus, when people are at risk of failing to cope in their own home, they need a range of help to cover a set of needs, both medical and social, that are particular to each person.

The project was therefore set up with three objectives:

1. To enable those elderly people who wished to continue living at home to do so, while improving their quality of life and general well-being.
2. To improve the effectiveness of socio-medical needs identification within the Primary Health Care Team (PHCT).
3. To enable PHCTs to provide or establish 'packages of care' appropriate to the identified needs of elderly people living at home.

The initial discussions between the Research Team and the Health Authority led to a proposal that focused on the organization of community care, identifying elderly people at risk and the importance of diagnosis and assessment. It outlined as the means of intervention a community Care Co-ordinator scheme. This was to involve a single person who would: first, act as a point of contact for the client; second, liaise with a multi-disciplinary team to help them devise an individual care package; and third, take responsibility for its implementation.

Evaluation

The Research Team considered (but rejected) a 'quasi-experimental' model for evaluation, preferring the greater flexibility and the detailed information about processes available through an 'action research' approach. The action research involved the development of new approaches (e.g. identifying elderly people at risk, assessing needs, setting up packages of care) in collaboration with existing service providers and evaluating them in the light of information from a variety of sources (monitoring data on individual cases, observational field data, and information from key informants including the care co-ordinators).

A detailed analysis of outcomes and costs was not undertaken. The Care Co-ordinator scheme was never intended as a model service which might simply replace existing services (although see Dant *et al* 1989 for a discussion of needs and the cost of providing co-ordination within the project).

The classic paradigm of comparing an experimental service with an existing service as a 'control' (see for example Challis and Davies 1986, Askham and Thompson 1990) was not used because it was felt that: (a) it would be unclear that a given outcome could be attributed to the particular style of intervention being developed; (b) the number of cases that were likely to be dealt with during the project would be too small for a persuasive sample size; and (c) the service intervention was being developed during the project and therefore could not be treated as a constant independent variable.

Most importantly, however, issues such as the role of information on local resources, the selection of techniques of assessment, the importance of collaborative working between professionals, and methods for co-ordinating and monitoring packages of care were the focus of the project rather than whether one service was better than another. Our purpose, then, was to learn about providing co-ordinated packages of care that could be implemented in service contexts in a variety of ways.

As it happened, the developing government policy (see Chapter 9, note 2) firmly shifted the lead responsibility for community care onto Social Services Departments towards the end of the Gloucester project. Combined with organizational changes within the health service (both sets of changes introduced through the National Health Service and Community Care Acts 1990), this meant that the findings of the project were unlikely to have any significant impact on services development within Gloucester or any other Health Authority. Nevertheless, we hope that the accounts of the processes involved in providing co-ordinated care contained in the Reports and Project Papers[1] from the Gloucester study and outlined in this chapter, will remain applicable in the changing context of providing community support for elderly people in Britain.

The Care Co-ordinators in the Gloucester Project

The Gloucester project was based on the provision of three keyworkers, called Care Co-ordinators, each attached to one of three PHCTs. There were three aspects to their role:

1. Gathering and exchanging information on services and resources available locally that may help elderly people to remain in their own homes for as long as possible;
2. Assessing the individual needs of elderly people who were patients of the practice and assisting in meeting those needs, by the co-ordination and monitoring of appropriate packages of care;
3. Gathering information for research purposes on the effect of services on individuals, and on the availability and appropriateness of services.

The Care Co-ordinators worked as members of the PHCTs, receiving referrals of individual cases from other members of the team (and occasionally from outside it) and sharing with them the specialist knowledge they were gathering on local facilities. On the basis of an assessment of the elderly person's needs, the Care Co-ordinator set up a 'package of care' linking statutory, voluntary and informal services to enable the elderly person to remain at home. Such a package might include, for example; nursing services, day care and other provision as well as 'buying in' private or local care. An important part of co-ordination was to link such services with the care being provided by relatives, friends and neighbours.

We have used the fashionable term 'package of care' because it distinguishes an approach that tries to address all of a person's needs from one that focuses on a single or limited dimension of care. It is, however, a misleading phrase in that it suggests something neat and tidy which can be handed over like consumer goods. As is well known by practitioners in the field of community care, providing care and support to meet elderly people's individual needs is not like that. Each package has to be tailored to fit that person, and each element of service, piece of equipment or source of informal support has to be carefully assessed, agreed upon and often tried out and re-negotiated for each package. In the Gloucester project it was found that this could be a continuous process sometimes lasting for a period of years. This can mean that the services and resources involved in the package of care have to be assessed, negotiated and co-ordinated several times.

Fulfilling the role as co-ordinators of care required undertaking a number of tasks which we have discussed more fully elsewhere (Dant and Gearing 1990). These tasks included the assessment of the person's needs, designing and setting up a package of care, and monitoring that package to ensure that it was meeting the person's needs. To be effective as a keyworker the Care Co-ordinators needed to know what local resources were available, and to develop a working relationship with other professionals providing services in the community.

As well as co-ordinating resources they were given small budgets so that they could use cash, not to buy in regular services but to buy one-off items of a 'taster' of a service. The Care Co-ordinator's own continuing involvement and relationship with the individuals on their caseloads was another resource which not only enabled them to monitor needs and re-negotiate them, but also became an important element in the service they offered to individuals. Care Co-ordinators provided advice (for example on welfare benefits, holidays, charities), personal counselling, and support (see Dant *et al* 1989 for a fuller account).

Within this pilot project the Care Co-ordinators had to undertake research tasks and seek out ways of meeting their own training needs. They also experienced complex lines of accountability, being employed by the Health Authority, working within the PHCT and having their role devised and altered by the Research Team.

Identifying Cases

One of the aims of the CEPH project was to develop an approach to identifying elderly people at risk. This issue has attracted concern since the high level of unreported medical and social needs amongst elderly people was demonstrated by Williamson and his colleagues (Williamson *et al* 1964). The Research Team carefully considered the literature on screening and case-finding but came to the conclusion that the advantages of such an approach were not warranted by the enormous investment of staff time (see Dant *et al* 1987). Instead, an 'opportunistic case-finding' approach was adopted in which the PHCT was encouraged to refer to the Care Co-ordinators elderly people 'at risk of failing to cope in their own homes'.

This approach was based on the very high proportion of elderly people who see their doctor in the course of a year (see for example Williams 1984). Within the CEPH project a retrospective study at the end of the first year showed that over 87% of patients aged over 75 had seen their general practitioner (GP) at least once during the previous year. The aim of the opportunistic case-finding approach was to take the opportunity of a contact for any other purpose to review how the patient over 75 was coping. To help the members of the PHCTs in considering whether someone was at risk, they were asked to consider a set of indicators drawn up by the Research Team on the basis of previous research and experience within the project (see Dant *et al* 1987). Five indicators were used:

1. Elderly people living with a carer or family any one of whom is showing signs of stress.
2. Elderly people with dementia or whose confusion may indicate dementia.
3. Elderly people under pressure to move from their home or who are giving up their home for any other reason.
4. Elderly people experiencing social isolation which is resulting in distress or depression.
5. Elderly people with significant health or social needs, who are refusing offers of service or support.

Continuity of contact with the practice population puts GPs in an excellent position for assessing that someone has more than medical needs. There was, however, a difference as to how doctors interpreted this more-than-just-medical role. Some saw themselves as a point of contact and referral, others felt that they had a more central role to play in co-ordinating services as well as in identifying the services that were needed. Viewing the doctor's role as broader than medical seems to be necessary if care co-ordination is to be usefully based on the PHCT; without it the identification of elderly patients at risk becomes a major task in itself.

Developing an Approach to Assessment

The assessment of someone's needs is an important precursor of providing any sort of support or care. What elderly people do and do not need, and indeed what they do and do not want, should determine what support is offered. The approach to assessing the multiple problems of elderly people at risk that was developed during the CEPH study was designed to take into account each person's individuality and particular circumstances. The person's present social situation was assessed in the context of their past life experience by the Care Co-ordinator. This approach attempted to get away from the tendency to offer a ready-made service response (such as home help or meals-on-wheels) and to work out with that person a 'solution' which fitted their individual needs and preferences. The detailed records that the Care Co-ordinators kept formed the basis of individual case studies (see Dant 1988, Boulton *et al* 1989, Dant *et al* 1989).

As well as developing a biographical approach to assessment, a systematic record of the elderly person's circumstances and needs was kept using a 'checklist' (see Dant *et al* 1987). This was a form with preset categories that was completed using information derived primarily from the elderly person but also from other sources including relatives, carers and the PHCT. Completing the checklist ensured that all aspects of a person's situation were considered during the assessment process. It incorporated a record of those needs that the elderly person had agreed with the Care Co-ordinator. The checklist was designed so that it could be used for monitoring at six-monthly intervals, with changes in both circumstances and needs noted.

The Biographical Approach

The biographical approach in the CEPH project started from a set of ideas which partly derived from previous research projects involving the collection of life histories which two of us (see Johnson 1976, Cornwell and Gearing 1989) had carried out, and partly from the literature on biography and life history. The principles from that research which seemed particularly relevant to assessment were:

- Those who listen to the life stories of older people whom they wish to help gain markedly different pictures of the person and their needs from those who administer traditional assessment techniques;
- Self-esteem can be greatly enhanced by skilful encouragement of reminiscence;
- The way people cope with the multiple losses associated with later life is directly dependent on earlier life experiences and on the remaining core of valued relationships, status roles and activities.

Early in the project we thought in terms of translating interview schedules that had been used in biographical research into some form of practitioner tool or codified assessment instrument (see Johnson *et al* 1988). The Care Co-ordinators tried out a number of different methods of assessment using life history interview schedules, a biographical record sheet, and a life-time chart to help with mapping people's life career.

Many of the early interviews were tape-recorded, transcribed and analysed by the project team. The aim was to develop an approach to assessment which reflected the principles mentioned above but which we could also demonstrate to be effective and efficient in a very practical context – the everyday practice of health care professionals. With the support of the Research Team the Care Co-ordinators worked on developing and refining the biographical approach to assessment during the three years of the project. Their location within the PHCT greatly facilitated this because they were able to draw on what was already known about the elderly patients both through colleague's memories and checking files. Moreover, they were able to compare the picture they developed of individual elderly people with that of the more function oriented view of colleagues in the PHCT. Early ideas and methods devised by the Research Team were considerably modified in the light of the Care Co-ordinators' actual experience of working with their older clients.

Care Co-ordinators learned that the biographical approach had to be used flexibly. For example, rather than pursuing a systematic and strictly chronological progression through the stages of someone's life from childhood onwards, they found it was more realistic to attend to presenting needs and then work back as opportunities allowed in the course of an interview, to discuss earlier experiences attitudes and relationships. Eventually, and in most cases, an acceptable way of meeting people's needs emerged. But this could vary in the time it took, from one or two lengthy sessions lasting a total of around an hour, to a less concentrated interaction in which different parts of the life history were disclosed and pieced together over several visits, during which other more immediate, or practical concerns were also discussed. Elsewhere (Boulton *et al* 1989) we have attempted to demonstrate how the biographical approach worked in practice through six lengthy case studies. The case studies and recorded biographical interviews are, we feel, the best evidence of the value of this approach to individuals. The appropriateness and usefulness of the biographical approach will vary from case to case but we have identified certain situations in which it has proved particularly useful:

- Eliciting older people's attitudes to a broad range of things and experiences (e.g. old age, life-style, interests, relationships, personal standards, services and residential care)
- Understanding family relationships
- Finding out about relationships between carers and the older person
- Discovering kinds of help, including services, which would be acceptable and unacceptable, with reference to providing a package of care
- Relating to and understanding people labelled 'difficult'
- Hearing how people coped with past difficulties and hardships with a view to how they might be helped in future crises
- Eliciting a different picture of people's needs
- Understanding and relating to people who suffer from dementia
- Helping people to get traumatic events into perspective
- Uncovering particular talents and aspirations which may suggest future activities

Putting the Biographical Approach into Practice

An important issue concerns how best to translate an action research experiment into the everyday practice of professionals. One conclusion we draw from the project is that it has to be done through a means which enables the worker to understand and feel comfortable with the *principles* of the biographical approach and of biographical interviewing, and to incorporate these into his or her style of working.

We have learnt that the biographical approach is very useful in assessing the needs of individual elderly people, and of finding acceptable ways of meeting those needs. However, it was used successfully in the project as a result of a sensitive and flexible application of the principles of biographical assessment by the Care Co-ordinators. Rather than strictly adhering to a pre-formulated set of methods and processes devised initially by the Research Team, the Care Co-ordinators adapted the approach to take into account the differing personalities and circumstances of their clients.

It is important to recognize, therefore, that the biographical approach to assessment is precisely that an *approach* which can be learnt, adapted, and employed in the light of particular circumstances and constraints which differ from one professional context to another. It is not a 'tool' which practitioners should be expected to apply rigidly. It follows that one legacy of the project could be an education and training programme for professionals in the principles and processes involved in the biographical assessment of older people, rather than a codification of a set of methods or procedures to be used indiscriminately by health and social work professionals. We believe that if used in this way the approach could be usefully adapted by a range of workers with older people in the health and social services.

The Cases

At the end of the first twelve months the Care Co-ordinators had received a total of 229 referrals and had taken on 143 people whom they felt were at risk and whom they could help. In the following twelve months they took on a further 29 cases making a total of 172 cases. During the two year period of recording information on these cases the caseloads fluctuated from a lowest figure of 15 to a highest of 47; the average caseload was 32.

A number of people were on the caseload for a long time; 56 of the 172 were cases for more than eighteen months of the two years, and 99 were cases for more than twelve months. The Care Co-ordinators only closed a case when there was clearly no more co-ordination work to be done. In practise this was when someone died, went permanently into institutional care, or moved from the area.

Each 'case' involved at least one elderly person but many also involved carers. There were seven elderly couples where both partners were 'cases' because both were at risk and needed co-ordinated care. Sometimes the carer was not the 'case' but received the support; here the elderly person who was the focus of care was the case for recording purposes. It is important to stress that while for the research requirement of systematic recording the concept of 'case' was appropriate, it was not the way in which the Care Co-ordinators thought or talked about the people they worked with. Each was a person with their own qualities, relationships, personal history and needs.

From the data gathered from monitoring instruments we are able to describe as a group the elderly people helped by the Care Co-ordinators. The 172 people who were cases were aged between 67 and 100 with a mean age of just under 80 at the time of their first meeting with the Care Co-ordinators. Overall, 25% of cases were men (see Figure 12.1). Most cases were referred either by the GP or the District Nurse but the Care Co-ordinators did receive a number of referrals from other sources (see Figure 12.2).

A 'diagnosis' or specific medical condition was not recorded as the aim was to assess the impact of people's state of health and well-being on their daily lives. For this reason the collection of health data focused on the functional problems (see Figure 12.3) and the ability to perform 'activities of daily living' (see Figure 12.4).

This group of elderly people were facing a number of problems in remaining at home and in many respects were more comparable to people living in residential accommodation than to people who received home care

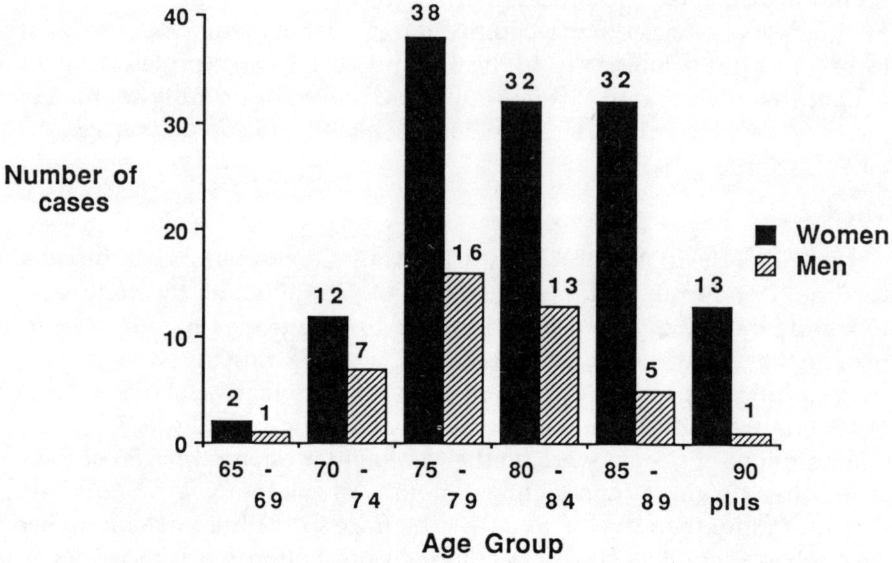

Figure 12.1: The CEPH Project: Distribution of all cases by age and sex

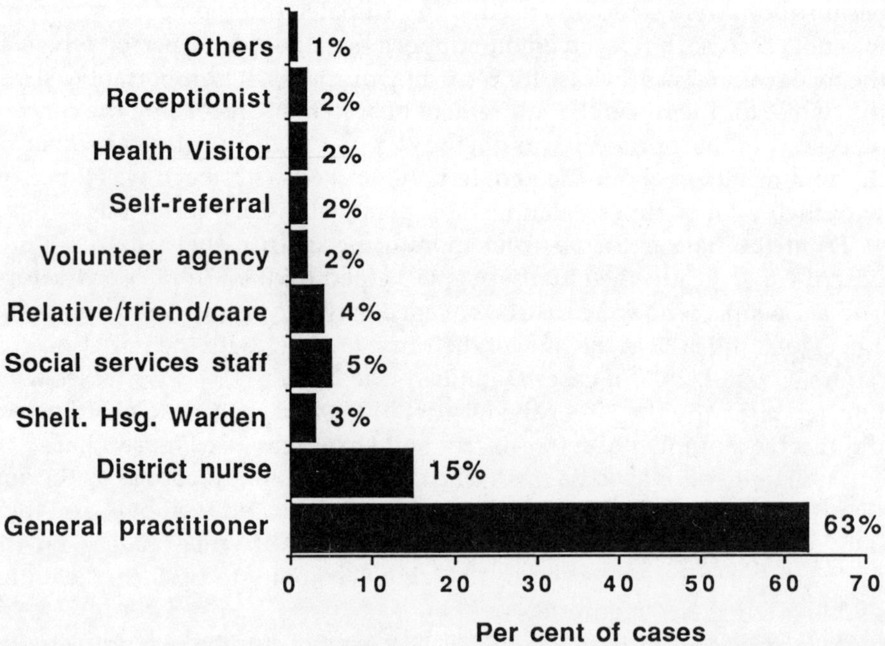

Figure 12.2: All cases: Sources of referral to care co-ordinators

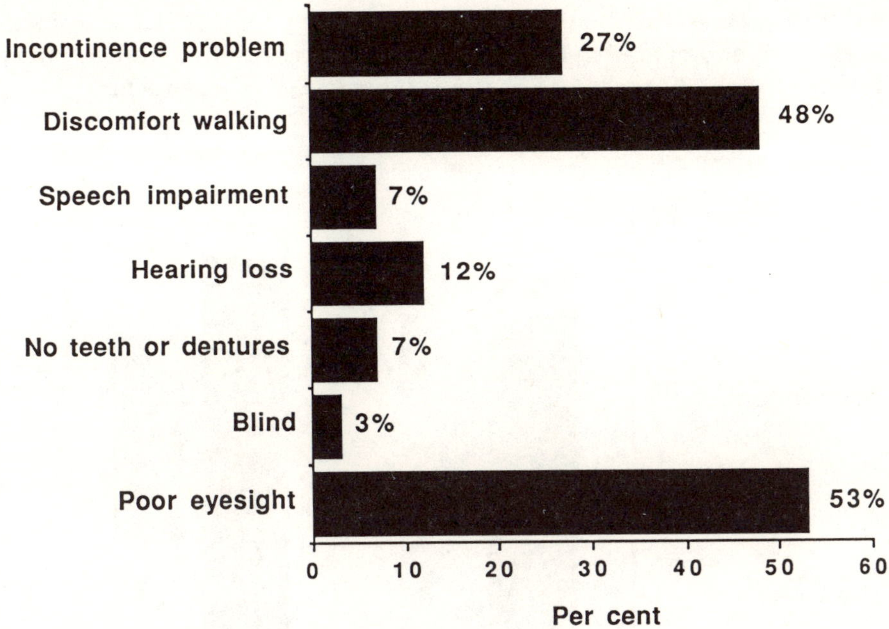

Figure 12.3: All cases: Distribution of functional problems recorded

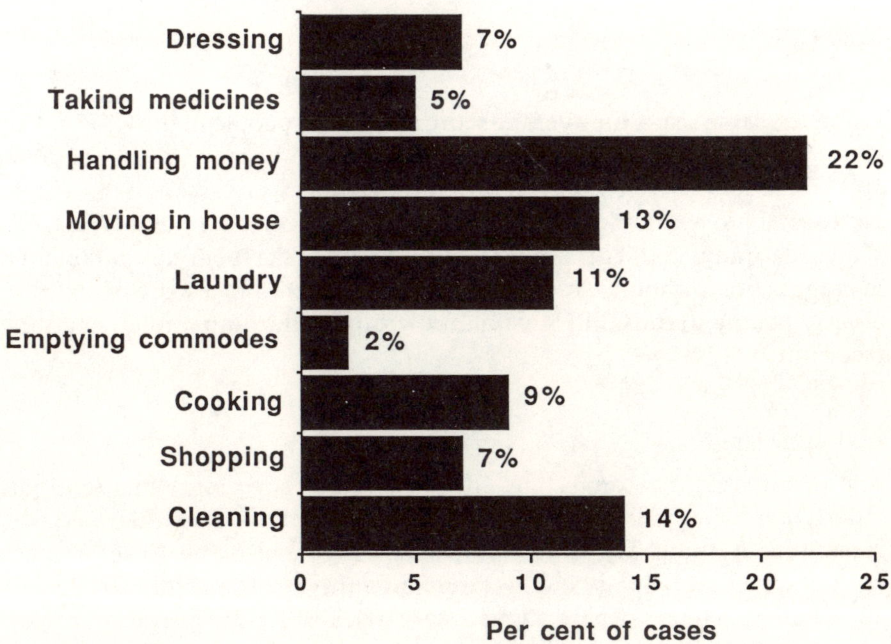

Figure 12.4: All cases: Needs related to activities of daily living

support. Using data from a study of 1023 residential care clients in Gloucestershire local authority homes, 'dependency scores' for CEPH and residential clients are compared in Figure 12:5. These scores resulted from a battery of items, with higher scores indicating higher levels of dependency.

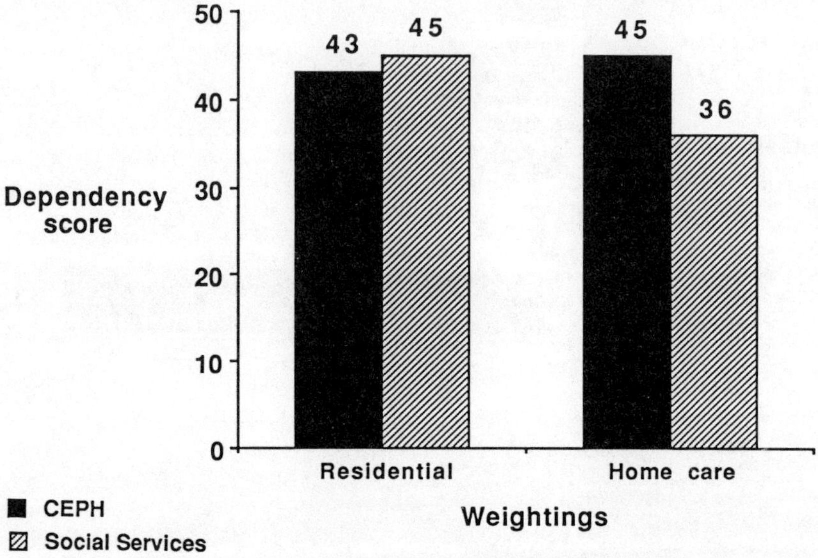

Figure 12.5: Comparison of dependancy scores between CEPH cases and Social Services clients

Using the same scale, the average score for elderly people in the CEPH study was 43. The scale was also used in a study of 406 home care clients (about 10% of the service's clients), but different weights were given to those items appropriate to assessing dependency in the home environment. The CEPH scores were adjusted with similar weightings to make them comparable. The average score for home care clients was 36 compared to a score of 45 for the elderly people in the CEPH evaluation group with comparable weightings (see Figure 12.5).

Meeting Needs

The action research project in Gloucester was successful in identifying elderly people at risk of institutionalization and it assessed their needs for remaining at home. The Care Co-ordinators were also able to set up packages of care that helped people to remain at home by meeting their needs. To monitor packages of care, for both research and service purposes, reviews of the assessment were held at six monthly periods. Of the 172 cases taken on during the project, 140 remained cases for long enough to receive at least one six monthly review. This group had 1092 needs identified at their initial assessment, some 794 of which had been met by the end of the evaluation period. Of course, within this group people were in contact with the Care Co-ordinator for different periods of time. The group diminished because people died, moved away or moved into residential forms of care. Also, people receiving their initial assessment later in the project not only had less time in which their needs could be met, but less time in which they could receive a review.

A consumer study with 96 cases, based on interviews either with the person who had been supported or their principal informal carer, showed that most (66%) felt that their support had either been better or much better as a result of the Care Co-ordinators involvement. Eighty per cent felt that the Care Co-ordinator had helped them to be clearer about their needs and 91% felt that the Care Co-ordinator had helped to meet their needs either 'well' or 'very well'. While the responses in consumer studies are notoriously difficult to interpret there seemed to be a general approval of the Care Co-ordinators' involvement. One thing that did emerge from the consumer study was that many people who had received support that had been organized by the Care Co-ordinator either did not remember in any detail about it or did not attribute to the Care Co-ordinator any role in its provision.

The Views of Other Practitioners

Practitioners in the PHCTs and the social services teams came to accept the Care Co-ordinators although there had been many misgivings about their role to begin with. The role of co-ordination was one that some individuals in different professions felt that they already undertook with the cases they were involved in (district nurses, social workers, general practitioners, occupational therapists, health visitors and home care organizers). There was some resentment of the Care Co-ordinators' intrusion into their responsibility and autonomy. Some professionals felt that what was needed were simply more direct resources.

However, other members of the same professional groups welcomed the Care Co-ordinators' contribution. In taking on responsibility for co-ordinating packages of care they left the professionals free to concentrate on the tasks they had been specifically trained for. The Care Co-ordinators developed an awareness of a range of resources available in their areas in the public, voluntary and private sectors that other professionals respected and appreciated. The members of the PHCTs all found value in the approach of care co-ordination though there was some variation of views about who should take on the role. Many of the professionals interviewed were enthusiastic about the approach and said that the Care Co-ordinators would be missed when the project ended and they withdrew.

It became clear as the Care Co-ordinators developed their role that other professionals were not aware of the range of resources available and had not been taking responsibility for establishing a package of care. There were examples of good liaison between services and of joint working to meet needs. But the assessment procedures of the various professional staff were primarily directed to their own input and only secondarily to other apparent needs of the person. The involvement of other sources of support was usually introduced by referring to the agency providing the support. The commitment to systematically establish a need for, introduce and then monitor a range of sources of support that together worked as a package was not characteristic of existing professional practice.

Conclusions

One of the things that did emerge quite clearly from the project was that the PHCT is a good locus for identifying elderly people at risk. The opportunistic case finding approach was extremely successful in identifying appropriate cases. While some referrals came from outside the PHCT, it was not always clear *exactly* where the referral originated; some may have been channeled through the GP although originating elsewhere while others came direct to the Care Co-ordinator but on the GP's advice. In the study of contact between GPs and their elderly patients at the end of the first year of referrals, those who had not seen the GP were contacted to find what proportion were at risk. Only five people were assessed as being at risk over the three practices (6% of those who had not seen the GP). This fitted with previous findings that those who do not see their GP are in generally good health (Williams 1984). Moreover, those people who do not see their GP are a relatively manageable group to follow up – far easier than a total screening approach.

What is perhaps more important is that the opportunistic case finding approach builds on the knowledge the PHCT have of their patients and encourages attention to the potentially broader needs of older people. The requirement of the 1990 contract[2] for GPs to offer a home assessment to people over 75 is likely to be interpreted by many as leading to a system of screening similar to that used to monitor child development. It could however be incorporated into normal practice and provide a first stage referral for a service that would undertake a comprehensive assessment of a person's needs and then co-ordinate care where appropriate.

The project also showed that there was considerable advantage in adopting a person centred approach to assessment. The rapport that developed between the Care Co-ordinators and the people they were working with enabled them to understand each person's needs individually. While the biographical approach could not be reduced to a systematic assessment tool, its value lay in alerting the Care Co-ordinator to those circumstances and aspects of history that provided the context of current needs. This meant that services or support that might otherwise be refused could be negotiated to fit the individual's needs. Adopting a biographical approach to assessment did not conflict with gathering systematic information on current needs through a checklist. The two approaches to assessment complemented each other and provided the basis of a comprehensive assessing, recording and monitoring system.

Finally, the project showed that elderly people at risk benefited from having an identified keyworker to co-ordinate their care. That is, someone involved in assessment, planning for support, establishing a 'package' of support, and monitoring it (see Dant and Gearing 1990, p.335). In the CEPH project the role of keyworker was filled by the Care Co-ordinator. However, some members of professions in the community already working with elderly people are well placed and keen to undertake this intensive keyworking role as an extension of their existing professional responsibilities (e.g. occupational therapists, home care organizers, social workers, district nurses, health visitors, community psychiatric nurses).

While there are advantages in introducing specialized staff to provide care co-ordination (it has been tried with considerable success in the Gloucester CEPH study and other projects) there are also disadvantages. It would mean, for example, introducing a large number of new posts which would be very expensive and would be unlikely to be more than a piecemeal development with the limited funds available to health and local authorities. Introducing specialist workers would also create a new, different professional to add to the already considerable number working with elderly people in the community. There is a danger that this would exacerbate the divisions between existing professional staff and services that make care co-ordination necessary, and confuse elderly people and their carers by having a new type of person to relate to. There is no technical speciality involved in care co-ordination although it does require good interpersonal and administrative skills, imagination and ingenuity. The three Care Co-ordinators in the Gloucester project came with different professional and work experiences (mixtures which included nursing, social work and teaching) which enabled them to develop the role. There was no reason to believe that any one of the professions currently working with elderly people in the community would be more suited to care co-ordination than any other. Training to undertake the tasks of a keyworker or Care Co-ordinator could be by in-service short courses building on existing professional training.

Within the CEPH project, the Care Co-ordinators acted as go-betweens linking the various services and professionals. While this was effective in meeting the needs of individual elderly people it did little or nothing to improve collaboration between the various services and professions. Because of this we did not recommend to Gloucester Health Authority that the way forward was to employ specialist Care Co-ordinators. Instead we suggested that they improve co-ordination amongst existing staff by convening multi-disciplinary teams in the community to identify elderly people at risk, assign keyworkers and set up packages of care. This would involve a high level of collaboration and commitment for existing workers and there would be good spin-off effects for those elderly people not at-risk and not receiving a package of care but perhaps needing more than one source of support.

Not all professionals are keen to take on this extra role, even with extra resources to enable them to do so. In these situations we recommended that a care co-ordination style post could be created, perhaps using funding through the Family Health Services Authority[3] in much the same way as general practitioners employ practice nurses. Overall we recommended a flexible approach. Care co-ordination is not a specialized professional task but it does require the adoption of certain strategies, and the co-operation of colleagues who actually control services.

Notes

1. In-house reports and papers relating to the Gloucester Project are available from: The Department of Health and Social Welfare, The Open University, Walton Hall, Milton Keynes, MK7 6AA.
2. From 1990, General Practitioners working within the National Health Service in Britain are obliged to offer a home assessment to all listed patients aged 75+. The assessment, covering aspects of mental and physical health, may be made by the GP, or by a delegated professional (e.g. Practice Nurse).
3. The Family Health Services Authority (FHSA) is an agency within the National Health Service responsible for the administration and co-ordination of local Primary Health Care.

References

Askham, J. and Thompson, C. (1990) *Dementia and Home Care: A Research Report on a Home Support Scheme for Dementia Sufferers.* London: Age Concern.

Boulton, J., Gully, V., Matthews, L. and Gearing, B. (1989) *Developing the Biographical Approach in Practice with Old People, Care for Elderly People at Home: Project Paper 7.* Milton Keynes: Open University.

Challis, D. and Davies, B. (1986) *Case Management and Community Care: An Evaluated Experiment in the Home Care of the Elderly.* Aldershot: Gower.

Cornwell, J. and Gearing, B. (1989) 'Doing Biographical Reviews with Older People'. *Oral History* 12 (1).

Dant, T. (1988) 'Old Poor and At Home: Social Security and Elderly People in the Community'. In Baldwin, S., Parker, G. and Walker R. (eds) *Social Security and Community Care.* Aldershot: Avebury.

Dant, T. and Gearing, B. (1990) 'Keyworkers for Elderly People in the Community: Case Managers and Care Co-ordinators'. *Journal of Social Policy* 19 (3): 331–360.

Dant, T., Carley, M., Gearing, B. and Johnson, M. (1987) *Identifying, Assessing and Monitoring the Needs of Elderly People at Home, Care for Elderly People at Home: Project Paper 2.* Milton Keynes: Open University.

Dant, T., Carley, M., Gearing, B. and Johnson, M. (1989) *Co-ordinating Care: The Final Report of the Care for Elderly People at Home Project, Gloucester.* Milton Keynes: Open University.

Johnson, M. (1976) 'That was your life: a biographical approach to later life'. In Munnichs, J.M.A. and Van den Heuval, W.J.A. (eds) *Dependency and Interdependency in Old Age.* The Hague: Martinus Nijhoff. Re-printed in Carver, V. and Liddiard, P. (1979) (eds) *An Ageing Population.* London: Hodder and Stoughton.

Johnson, M., Gearing, B., Carley, M. and Dant, T. (1988) *A Biographically Based Health and Diagnostic Technique: A Research Report, Care for Elderly People at Home: Project Paper 4.* Milton Keynes: Open University.

Williams, E.I. (1984) 'Characteristics of patients over 75 not seen during one year in general practice'. *British Medical Journal* 291, 251–254.

Williamson, J., Stokoe, I.H., Gray, S., Fisher, M. and Smith, A. (1964) 'Old people at home; their unreported needs'. *The Lancet* 1, 1117–1120.

CHAPTER 13

The Effect of the Social Environment on Demented Elderly People in Residential Care

Ann Netten

Wagner (1988) took it as a point of principle that a move into residential care should be a 'positive choice'. Choice implies a level of knowledge about the likely outcomes of different options. From very early on in the study of residential care of elderly people (e.g. Townsend 1962, Barton 1966) there has been a conviction among researchers, observers and practitioners alike that the social environment of homes must have a profound effect on the quality of life of the residents. Translating this belief into clearly identified and tested hypotheses has proved an elusive task, however. It is a task that encounters particular difficulties when the residents concerned are suffering from dementia.

This paper briefly reviews and discusses the principal approaches to the assessment of the social environment and identifies where these have been applied to the residential care of people with dementia. The results of a study which used two of these approaches to examine the effect of the social environment on outcomes for such residents are then described.

Caring Regimes

Much of the work concerned with assessing social environments in residential care has concentrated on the classification of the social environment of homes for elderly people in terms of caring regimes. The aim has been to define and measure aspects of care practices and policies that are assumed to have negative or beneficial effects. In defining these effects several studies have drawn on Goffman's (1961) theory of total institutions (e.g. Hughes and Wilkin 1980). A 'total institution' is one in which:

1. all aspects of daily life are conducted in the same place under the same authority;
2. daily activity is carried out with large numbers of others who are treated alike and doing the same thing;

3. daily activity is routinised and fixed to a schedule which is imposed on inmates by formal rulings and a body of officials; and
4. the various enforced activities and routines constitute 'a rational plan' designed to fulfil the official aims of the institution.

In this theoretical structure the outcome for residents is represented as institutionalization or excessive dependency. For example, Booth (1985) states that increased dependency was seen as a likely outcome in that 'the weight of informed opinion now accepts that the process of care may in itself induce dependency'. Similarly, Baltes, Burgess and Stewart (1980) showed that staff in USA nursing homes typically failed to respond to independent behaviour but strongly supported dependent behaviour.

Booth (1985) used cluster analysis on data collected to reflect the regimes of homes. He identified three clusters of homes, which he defined as having positive, mixed or restrictive regimes (see Table 13.1). Although this provided a useful way of categorizing homes, the different types of home did not appear to affect the outcome for residents in terms of dependency indicators (Booth 1986).

Table 13:1 Booth's regime types

Positive	Homes which tend to allow residents to do or decide things for themselves, leaving them a greater area of freedom of action and individual choice.
Mixed	Homes with multiple regimes, opportunities for freedom and choice in some areas and not others and those whose approach consistently fell between the other two groups.
Restrictive	Homes that tend to adopt a narrow or restrictive view of residents' capabilities, limiting freedom of action and denying opportunities for deciding things for themselves.

A methodology devised by King, Raynes and Tizard (1971) to evaluate homes for people with mental handicaps was adapted by Kimbell, Townsend and Bird (1974) for use in old people's homes. Institutions were classified as tending towards resident-oriented or institutionally-oriented regimes along four dimensions: rigidity of routine; block treatment; depersonalization; and social distance between staff and inmates. Again, no relationship was found between overall dependency and regime but the level of mental confusion among residents was related to low social distance between staff and residents and a more structured routine. One of the problems of such a cross-sectional study, is difficulty in establishing cause and effect. For example, the officers-in-charge who provided a more flexible routine may have been more prepared to admit and tolerate confused residents.

Another cross-sectional study of six homes in depth also used the King, Raynes and Tizard (1971) methodology and observational techniques to assess homes that had a mixture of confused and lucid residents (Evans *et al* 1981). In this study engagement and the views of residents were used as indicators of the effects of the physical and social environments. This found that rigid traditional definitions of staff roles were associated with poor staff relations, which were in turn associated with lower levels of activity and social interaction among residents. The principal result of this study was, however, that above a certain level (about a third) a higher proportion of confused residents had a detrimental effect on care practices.

Methodologies that base the assessment of regimes on enumerating care policies and practice encounter a number of problems. The 'regime' of a home may be inconsistent; Booth *et al* (1982) argue that in many homes there are multiple regimes – that homes are a confused mixture of unnecessary, unhelpful rules and sensitive practice. Moreover, the indicators chosen may not be empirically consistent in reflecting the desired aspect of the home. Clarke and Bowling (1990) found that observation techniques revealed variations in caring regimes not evident from survey techniques for assessing the 'totality' of regimes.

Many of the terms used in these investigations are heavily value laden. Regimes are 'positive' if they allow greater freedom. Regimes are 'restrictive' if they limit choice. Residents are described as 'victims' and so on. Such labelling may not be appropriate, particularly in the care of people with dementia. Hegeman and Tobin (1988) conducted a survey of autonomy enhancement programmes for mentally impaired elderly people in the three states in the USA. They found a number of programmes which were described as autonomy enhancing but involved the use of locked and segregated units. Several of these reported enhanced functioning of residents. The authors suggest this is due to elimination of other physical or chemical restraints which may ultimately increase functioning and authentic decision making. It may be inappropriate, therefore, to label certain practices or policies as 'restrictive' or 'positive' without a clear association with the outcomes for the residents.

Ecological and Psychological Approaches

An alternative transactional approach to the measuring of the social environment was developed by Kleemier (1961) who defined the regimes of facilities for elderly people by using three continuums: segregation/non-segregation; institutional control/non-institutional control; congregation/non-congregation. Pincus' (1968) work was based on this and distinguished four dimensions of the institutional environment: public/private; structured/unstructured; resource rich/sparse; and isolated/integrated. The measurement of each was done in terms of physical plans – rules and regulations, programmes, and staff behaviour – providing a set of 'cells' which describe the home. A fifth dimension – personalization – referring to social distance between staff and residents was added later (Pincus and Wood 1970).

The congruence model (Kahana, Liang and Felton 1980) drew both upon Kleemier and upon the ecological tradition in which human behaviour was represented as a function of the relationship between individuals and their environment. Morale in this model was predicted by measuring the 'fit ' between the elderly person and his or her environment. Congruence was measured on seven dimensions: segregation; congregation; institutional control; structure; stimulation; affect; and impulse control. In a study of three homes it was found that if there was too much congregate activity for the individual this would adversely affect morale. Similarly, morale was affected if the resident felt 'out of step' in whatever direction as regards 'impulse control'. However, it is worth noting that in the home in which individual-environmental congruence was least important, there were more options open to residents and the home had fewer 'total institution' features.

While this theoretical approach is very appealing, it runs into a number of difficulties if the intention is to assess residents with dementia. It presupposes an ability to know or to interpret the individuals' needs from their environment. To deduce these needs when the residents have senile dementia would require generalizations from their past histories, generalizations from characteristics of the condition across individuals and/or deductions from their current behaviour. All of these are likely to encounter validity problems which would be compounded by the difficulties in measuring outcomes such as environmental 'fit'.

The social ecology model (see for example Lawton 1974; 1979; 1982, Moos 1976, Moos and Lemke 1985) of aging provides a more fruitful approach as the outcomes are measured in behavioural and competence changes in individuals. The effect of environmental demands or 'press' depends upon the mental and physical competence of the individual. Too great a press or too little will lead to maladaptive behaviour. How the resident perceives this press (cognitive appraisal) will depend on both the external environment and the residents' competence and will in turn affect how residents deal with it (coping response). Coping responses in residential care would include engagement, territorial behaviour, way finding and so on. Each of these factors (personal competence, environmental influences, cognitive appraisal and coping responses) will affect in turn long term stability and change in the residents' abilities and behaviour patterns. The social ecology approach incorporates the environmental docility hypothesis in which 'the less competent the individual, the greater the impact of environmental factors on that individual' (Lawton 1982, p.14).

This would seem a particularly appropriate model in the measurement of the impact of the social environment on demented residents of homes for elderly people. A major difficulty that people with dementia have is negotiating and dealing with their environment. Their reduced competence clearly increases their vulnerability to environmental influences. Moreover, the emphasis in the social ecology approach on behavioural outcomes provides a practical solution to the problems of measuring outcomes such as 'morale' or 'fit'.

The Multiphasic Environmental Assessment Procedure (MEAP) was developed by Moos and Lemke (1984) as a method of assessing residential care settings. It is based on the social ecology model of aging and represents the different dimensions of the environmental system as interactive. It consists of a general rating scale, a checklist of physical and architectural

Table 13:2 Sheltered Care Environment Scale (SCES) subscale descriptions and item examples

Relationship Dimensions	
1. Cohesion	Measures how helpful and supporting staff members are towards residents and how involved and supportive residents are with each other. (e.g., Do residents get a lot of individual attention?)
2. Conflict	Measures the extent to which residents express anger and are critical of each other and of the facility. (e.g., Do residents ever start arguments?)
Personal Growth Dimensions	
3. Independence	Assesses how self-sufficient residents are encouraged to be in their personal affairs and how much responsibility and self-direction they are encouraged to exercise. (e.g., Do residents sometimes take charge of activities?)
4. Self Exploration	Measures the extent to which the residents are encouraged to openly express their feelings and concerns. (e.g., Are personal problems openly talked about?)
System Maintenance and Change Dimensions	
5. Organization	Assesses how important order and organisation are in the facility, the extent to which residents know what to expect in their day-to-day routine, and the clarity of rules and procedures. (e.g., Are activities for residents carefully planned?)
6. Resident Influence	Measures the extent to which the residents can influence the rules and policies of the facility and the degree to which the staff direct the residents through regulations. (e.g., Are suggestions made by the residents acted upon?)
7. Physical Comfort	Taps the extent to which comfort, privacy, pleasant decor and sensory satisfaction are provided by the physical environment. (e.g., Can residents have privacy whenever they want?)

Source: Moos and Lemke (1984)

features, a policy and programme information form, and a resident and staff information form. The Sheltered Care Environment Scale (SCES), which forms part of the MEAP, is designed to assess the character or social climate of a facility. Table 13.2 describes the seven dimensions of the social climate which comprise the SCES: cohesion; conflict; independence; self-exploration; organization; resident influence; and physical comfort. These are derived from 63 items which reflect the perceptions of all, or a proportion of the staff and residents in a facility.

This method of assessing the social environment represents a broader approach than the assessment of caring regimes identified above. Different climates will result from the characteristics of the resident population of the homes as well as the policies and practices of the care staff. The 'objective' information gathered by the policy and programme information form in the MEAP is closer in some ways to the basis of the regime measures. However, there is likely to be a close relationship between the regime and the social climate of a home: it might be possible to deduce the regime from the social climate. For example, low 'independence' and low 'resident influence' might reflect Booth's definition of a 'restrictive' regime. However, it would be impossible in the absence of numerous value laden assumptions to deduce from the regime types such aspects of the social climate as the level of 'cohesion' or 'conflict'.

Researchers have used parts and combinations of the MEAP as a basis both for assessing the social climate in different facilities and comparing facilities over time (e.g. Lemke and Moos 1980; 1981). This latter may be of particular interest when the intention is to effect change by changing the environment. A study by Ransen (1981) indicated that long term results of two intervention programmes were dependent on whether systematic alterations had occurred from a social ecological perspective. In examining determinants of the social climate Moos and Igra (1980) found that establishments with more socio-recreational activities and policies which encouraged resident control had high levels of 'cohesion' and 'independence'. Less 'resident influence' and 'independence' were found to be associated with higher staffing levels, even after allowance had been made for type of facility.

There is a wealth of research material and theories relating both to normal aging and the environment of institutions (e.g. Willcocks, Peace and Kellaher 1987), but much of the research into the particular difficulties of people with dementia has tended to focus on individual treatment programmes such as reality orientation. Environmental effects may have a fundamental influence on the outcome of such programmes (see for example Woods and Britton 1985) but relatively little research has focused on the effect of the environment of institutions as a whole on such residents. Those studies that have examined the institutional care of elderly people with dementia (e.g. Evans *et al* 1981; Norman 1987) have provided valuable insights but have not related these to outcomes for the demented residents themselves. Studies using the social ecological approach have used as outcomes other measures in MEAP such as resident functioning or community integration. The study reported here aims to contribute to the continuing debate on the most appropriate way forward in the residential care of demented elderly people by examining the relationship between the environment and individually measured outcomes for a sample of 'confused' residents.

Study Design

Thirteen homes for elderly people were selected from four local authorities: one inner and two outer London boroughs and one county. The homes and the residents in this study were not representative of homes and residents in the country as a whole. In particular, to enable a proper assessment of specialist provision, the study included a high proportion of specialist homes: 6 of the 13. As a result the population of the homes overall was more dependent than residents in care generally. Similarly, although the staffing levels were close to national levels there was a higher proportion of qualified staff, particularly with a nursing background. For each of the homes, officers-in-charge or senior staff completed a form based upon that used in the Personal Social Services Research Unit (PSSRU) survey of residential care (Darton 1983) which provided basic background and ability information for all residents. The intention was for ten residents to be selected from each home. The criteria on which they were selected were designed to allow comparability and to exclude such influences as the relocation effect. On this basis a sample of 104 residents were identified, all of whom had been assessed as moderately or severely confused, had been in the home for six months and were at least partially sighted.

The sample residents were assessed at the beginning and the end of a six month period using the Clifton Assessment Procedures for the Elderly (CAPE; Pattie and Gilleard 1979). Table 13.3 shows destinational outcomes for the sample residents: 79 residents in all survived this period in the home. Assessments of the environmental characteristics of the homes were made at the beginning of the six months by observation, interviewing senior staff and self report questionnaires for care staff.

Table 13:3 Number and level of confusion of residents in the study

	Level of Confusion		
	Moderate (n)	*Severe (n)*	*Total (n)*
Remained in the home	38	41	79
Transferred	4	3	7
Died	7	11	18
Total	49	55	104

Source: As assessed by senior staff member

Assessing the Social Environment

It has been argued (Bond et al 1989) that in addressing such a complicated issue as the process of residential care there is a need for methodological pluralism. In this study two approaches to assessing the social environment were adopted: to use the SCES developed by Moos and Lemke and to adopt a similar method to Booth and ask of senior members of staff a series of questions designed to identify normal care practices and policies.

The problem in using the latter approach in devising scales for 'privacy' or 'regimentation' is that these are likely to be applied in a very different way to 'confused' residents than to alert residents. Moderately or severely confused residents tend to be the exception rather than the rule. For example, Table 13.4 shows a variety of questions that it had been hoped might be used to devise such scales. These were asked both of the home as a whole and for each resident. If the answers to the questions asked for individual residents reflected the policy of the homes in which they were resident it would be anticipated that for each question the proportion of expected positive responses would be approximately equal to the reported individual response.

The responses demonstrate that the social environment experienced by a demented elderly person might be a very different experience indeed to that described for the home as a whole by a senior member of staff. For example, while the policy in all the homes was to allow residents free use of the grounds, in practice only 27% of the sample residents were allowed such freedom. Although all of the homes had gardens, only 4 of the 13 had an outside area that was enclosed and secure. This meant that considerations of safety resulted in restrictions on residents' movements.

Table 13:4 Contrast between the home and individual response to questions concerning home environment

	'Yes' Responses home policy (%)	*'Yes' Responses for sample residents (%)*
Chooses new clothes?	100	71
Allowed free use of grounds of home?	100	27
Chooses daily clothing?	95	64
Is bathed at time set by staff?	76	100
Gets up at time set by staff?	72	100
Allowed out of home unsupervised?	58	6
Goes to bed at time set by staff?	10	31

Sometimes the difficulties presented by residents resulted in a more flexible rather than restrictive caring strategies. For example, in one home residents were normally not allowed in their bedrooms for a certain period in the day. One particular demented resident in the home, however, rarely, if ever, left her room.

In evaluating the effect of the social environment on demented people it is of importance, therefore, both to measure the way the care practices impinge upon the individual and the overall social climate. Thus, in analysing outcomes, individual practice, such as set bedtimes, were used to indicate the individual's experience of care policies. For indicators of the overall social climate of the home it was decided to use Moos and Lemke's Sheltered Care Environment Scale (SCES). The advantages of the social ecology model of aging in this context have already been discussed. In addition a methodological advantage of the SCES is that it is compiled from forms completed by all members of care staff. Thus a composite view of the establishment is built up, rather than the specific view of one staff member.

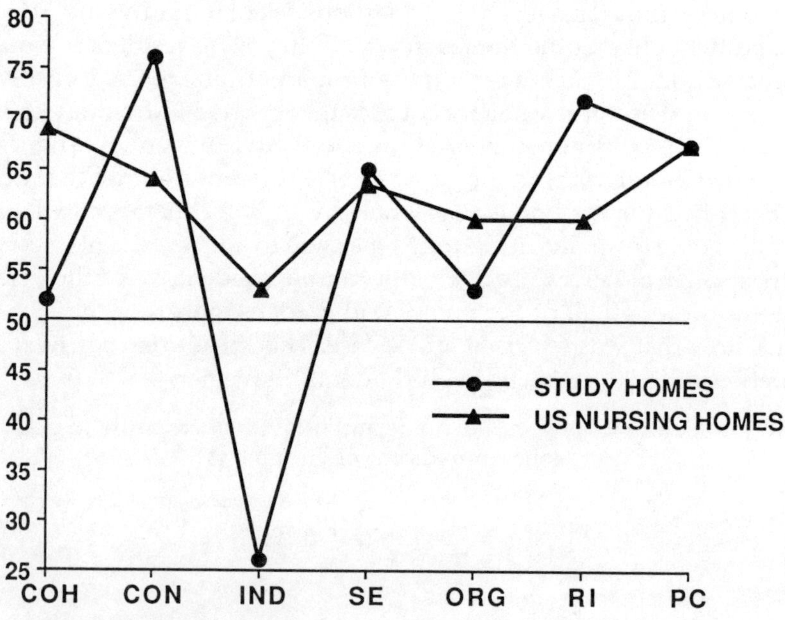

Figure 13.1: SCES scales: Study homes and US norms

Although the SCES scales provide useful indicators of individual aspects of the social climate, for a more general description of the homes Moos and Lemke use the concept of a home profile. Figure 13.1 demonstrates the profiles of the study and US nursing homes. Nursing homes were chosen to contrast with the study homes as the dependency characteristics of the residents were similar.

It is interesting to note the very different profiles of US nursing homes and the UK study homes. In particular, the relative values of the relationship sub-scales of cohesion and conflict are completely reversed with conflict, very high in contrast to the normative US levels. What appears of more concern, however, is the lower level of independence in the study homes. These included some with a very positive attitude to caring for elderly people and it seems unlikely that they are much worse on this dimension than UK homes as a whole. Resident influence is perceived by staff as higher in the study homes than in the US nursing homes, so UK homes may not compare in quite such a negative way with US homes as first appears. It would, however, be interesting to establish the residents' view of such aspects of the social environment.

Classification of Homes by Regime Type

Although the profiles provide useful descriptive devices for comparing groups of homes, it was felt that there was a need for some way of classifying the homes, in terms of their regime type or social climate profile. This should provide both a descriptive device and a tool in further analysis. In describing types of regime it is useful to refer to three types of regime identified by Booth (1985): positive, mixed and restrictive (see Table 13.1).

If this basis for describing the regimes is to be used in a classification using the SCES sub-scales, the most important sub-scales to be clearly defined are those of independence and resident influence. However, with the exception of physical comfort, all the dimensions of the social climate were used to determine the groups. In order to see whether the homes fell into regime types, cluster analysis was used as a purely exploratory technique. The clusters were examined when there were two to six clusters inclusive, to see if a pattern could be distinguished.

The initial division into two clusters appeared to divide the homes subsequently classified as homes with 'positive' regimes from the rest. Subsequent clusters, however, did not quickly identify a third group of 'restrictive' regimes. Initially specific homes were identified as outliers from the initial two groups.

A single home formed a separate group once three clusters were identified. The Officer-in-Charge left this home during the six months following the assessment and it was noticeable that cohesion and organization were significantly lower ($p<.05$) in this home than in the other homes in the study. This could be described as a 'stressed' profile and adds to the credibility of the use of the scales as a device for assessing the social climate. The SCES dimension scores on independence and resident influence indicated that overall this home fell into the 'mixed' type of regime. Another single home, once four clusters were identified, formed a separate group reflecting a difference in the way this positive regime was generated. This home had a very devolved structure using key workers in the decision making process. Thus organization was very much lower than in the other 'positive' homes where the personality of the officer-in-charge appeared to be working to motivate other staff in generating the positive, professional regime. Although this is obviously of interest, it was felt that the type of regime, higher independence, resident influence, cohesion and so on, should be the principal divide, rather than how this was achieved.

Three homes were variously grouped together using different methods of cluster analysis once five or six clusters were specified. In defining regime types, these homes were grouped together because the average scores for the sub-scales of independence and resident influence appeared to reflect the 'restrictive' type of regime.

Description of Regime Groupings

Table 13.5 shows the average and range of scores for each of the SCES dimensions. This demonstrates that the clusters of homes are well separated in those dimensions (independence and resident influence) which were identified at the outset as of importance in distinguishing 'positive' and 'restrictive' homes from the others. In addition the difference between the average scores between the groups were statistically significant for cohesion, organization and self-exploration.

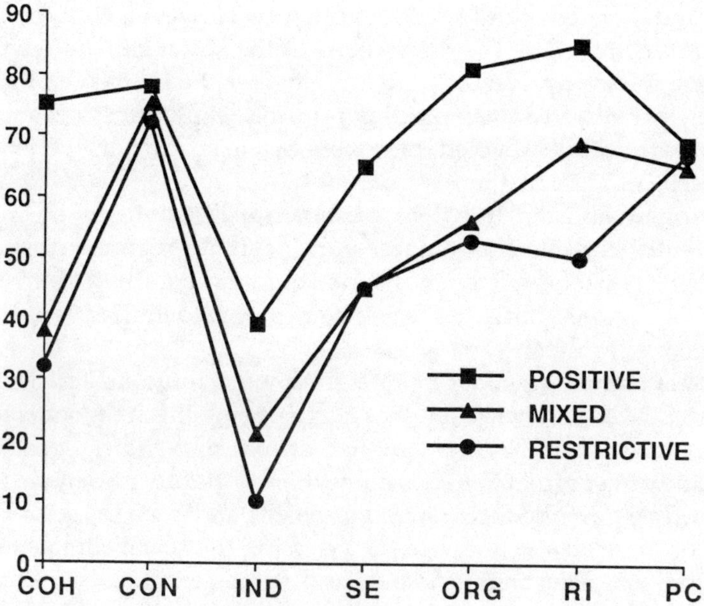

Figure 13.2: SCES Scales: Types of regime

The positive regimes were easily defined using the cluster analysis and Figure 13.2 shows that the profile of the homes with 'positive' regimes is noticeably different to that of the other types of home. In particular, cohesion is much higher, and at a similar level to conflict. Both the levels and the profile of the dimensions are closer to the US profile of nursing homes

(Figure 13.1) although independence is lower and resident influence higher, than in the US facilities. The homes which had 'restrictive' regimes were not so clearly defined in terms of the cluster analysis, however, and their profile in Figure 13.2 is less easily distinguished from the homes which were classified as having 'mixed' regimes.

Obviously, further work would need to be done over a larger sample of homes to establish both normative levels and measures of concurrent validity but this provides at least a starting point for developing a usable measure. For example, if the results of the study were validated by further research then one way of defining regimes of homes would be that a home scoring over 30 for independence *and* over 80 for resident influence could be defined as having a positive regime. If a home scored less than 12 on independence it would be regarded as having a restrictive regime.

Effect of Regime on Outcomes

The ultimate outcome or final output of a service is the welfare of the client or resident but a reliable measure of welfare for demented people has yet to be identified. One of the advantages of the social ecology approach identified earlier was that outcomes are defined in terms of changes in behaviour and competence. This model was modified for use in the study and the measures of outcome were all indicators of change over time using the CAPE scales (i.e., change in the level of socially disturbed behaviour, change in the level of apathy, and change in the level of orientation).

In using measures of change over a six month period the intention was to identify the effect of environmental factors on the resident rather than which types of environment and resident are associated. The latter can reflect policies of admission as much as causal effects but there is a major difficulty with using two time periods: there are inevitably people for whom no information is available at the second stage of the study. This may be because they have died, have been transferred, or are in hospital. In this study there was also one refusal of interview at the second stage (the lady thought the interviewer was from the police). The charge can be made that the results will therefore be biased, there may be a fundamental difference between the survivors and non-survivors.

The assumption made for the current analysis was that over a six month period death and temporary hospitalization could be seen to be random. It is less reasonable, however, to assume this for long term hospitalization and transfer to other establishments. Such moves may reflect a lower level of tolerance for certain behaviours by some establishments or a negative effect upon the resident resulting in more serious decline. Thus a non-random distribution of non-survivors would be expected. Only five people or 4.8% of the sample fell into this category, so given the assumption of random death and illness resulting in hospital admission (20 cases in all) this source of bias would appear limited.

Table 13:5 Distinguishing regime types

	Positive			*Mixed*			*Restrictive*		
	Max	*Min*	*Mean*	*Max*	*Min*	*Mean*	*Max*	*Min*	*Mean*
Cohesion* (51.6)	81.7	55.6	75.4	48.9	18.5	37.7	51.1	20.6	32.9
Conflict (75.8)	87.3	71.4	77.6	85.2	67.8	75.7	75.5	68.9	72.6
Independence* (25.5)	51.6	31.0	38.4	27.2	13.6	21.3	10.2	8.9	9.9
Organisation* (52.5)	71.4	46.0	65.0	58.9	18.5	44.1	51.1	38.4	44.7
Self-expression* (64.8)	86.1	60.3	80.6	58.3	51.1	55.4	56.5	44.4	52.7
Resident influence* (70.9)	90.5	81.7	85.9	74.4	56.1	68.2	51.4	44.4	48.8
Physical comfort (66.7)	74.6	55.6	68.0	69.1	53.7	64.9	76.9	53.3	66.7

Source: Figures in brackets refer to average scores
Significance levels refer to analysis of variance (F statistic) of scales.
* $p<.01$

A small number of variables were entered into the equation initially on theoretical grounds. These were the Time 1 level of the outcome variable, an indicator of depression and the length of stay in the home. The amount of change likely, or even possible given the restricted nature of the scales, depends on the initial level of the outcome variable. Depression can affect the prognosis of dementia symptoms (Rabins, Merchant and Nestadt 1984). The length of time the resident had been exposed to the environment of the home or 'treatment' will also affect changes in orientation and behaviour.

Variables were then allowed to enter in two stages using stepwise analysis. The first set included 'personal system' variables indicating abilities or competence and personal influences such as age. This was in order to allow for these influences before examining the environmental effects, both direct and indirect (e.g. the ability of the resident to find his or her way around the home). It is not practicable in this context to discuss fully the results of the analysis. The results showed that staff played a vital role in directly affecting outcomes for residents, but here the main interest is in how the staff and resident influences were captured in the measurement of the social environment and caring regimes.

The method of identifying a 'positive' regime appeared to gain credibility from the resulting analyses. It was associated with a beneficial influence on all three of the outcome measures: apathy ($b = -0.78$, $t = -2.16$, $p<.01$), social disturbance ($b = -0.88$, $t = -2.20$, $p<.01$) and orientation ($b = 0.59$, $t = 1.84$,

$p<.05$). Restrictive regimes did not appear to be associated with specific outcomes for residents and were less clearly defined as a grouping in the cluster analysis. One interpretation of this result is that residential care is, as a process, restrictive on residents. It requires a well defined positive set of values among the staff to counteract this process, to develop a positive attitude to the residents that feeds through to increased well being defined in behavioural and competence terms.

Of the individual indicators of caring regimes only one association was found. Residents showed less social disturbance at the end of the six month period if choosing what to wear each day was part of their normal routine ($b = -0.77$, $t = -2.2$, $p<.01$). It had been anticipated that this would provide an indicator of the level of control that residents were allowed over their lives. The result would suggest that absence of control increases frustration and antisocial behaviour.

Conclusion

With the increased emphasis upon consumer choice in the delivery of social care services there is a particular responsibility laid upon local authorities and health authorities in caring for people with mental health difficulties. The ability and credibility of such people in exercising choice or complaints systems are clearly curtailed. More than most they will be dependent upon effective inspection and quality assurance procedures. It is important that these are based soundly upon investigations which measure outcomes for the residents themselves.

If the results of the study reported here are confirmed, there is a potential in the use of the SCES scale and the assessment of 'positive' regimes. With such a small number of homes, however, the use of such measures must remain speculative, until larger studies have confirmed the method of assessing the regime and the impact on residents. The method of identifying a 'positive' regime gained credibility from the analyses of outcomes for the sample residents: a beneficial influence was associated with all three of the outcome measures: apathy, social disturbance and orientation. Such a comprehensive effect on the outcome measures argues for a relationship between this definition of a positive regime and the overall welfare of the demented residents.

Acknowledgements

My thanks go to all the staff and residents of the homes for their help and co-operation in this study and to David Challis and Ann Clewer for their advice and support.

References

Barton, R. (1966) *Institutional Neurosis, 2nd Ed.* Wright: Bristol.

Baltes, M., Burgess, R. and Stewart, R. (1980) 'Independence and dependence in self-care behaviours in nursing home residents: an operant-observation study'. *International Journal of Behavioural Development* 3, 489–500.

Benjamin, L. and Spector, J. (1990) 'Environments for the Dementing'. *International Journal of Geriatric Psychiatry* 5, 15–24.

Bond, J., Bond, S., Donaldson, C., Greyson, B. and Atkinson, A. (1989) 'Evaluation of an Innovation in the Continuing Care of Very Frail Elderly People'. *Ageing and Society* 9 (4) 347–381.

Booth, T. (1985) *Home Truths, Old Peoples Homes and the Outcome of Care.* Gower: Aldershot.

Booth, T. (1986) 'Institutional Regimes and Induced Dependency in Homes for the Aged'. *The Gerontologist* 26 (4) 418–423.

Booth, T., Barritt, A., Berry, S., Martin, D., Melotte, C., Phillips, D. (1982) 'A Confused Mixture'. *Community Care,* 2/12/82.

Clarke, P. and Bowling, A. (1990) 'Quality of Everyday life in Long Stay Institutions for the Elderly: An Observational Study of Long Stay Hospital and Nursing Home Care'. *Social Science and Medicine* 30, (11) 1201–1210.

Darton R.D. (1983) *Residential Accommodation for the Elderly 1970–81, PSSRU Discussion Paper 277/2. University of Kent at Canterbury.*

David, T., Moos, R. and Kahn, J. (1981) 'Community integration among elderly residents of sheltered care settings'. *American Journal of Community Psychology* 9 (5) 513–526.

Evans, G., Hughes, B., Wilkin, D., Jolley, D. (1981) *The Management of Mental and Physical Impairment in Non-specialist Residential Homes for the Elderly,* Research Report. Psychogeriatric Unit. University Hospital of South Manchester.

Fyvie, C. and Gledhill, K. (1989) *Measuring Staff Perceptions of Residential Care Settings for the Elderly,* Paper given at British Society of Gerontology Conference, Nottingham.

Goffman, E. (1961) *Asylums: Essays on the Social Situation of Mental Patients and other Inmates:* Garden City, New York: Anchor Books.

Hegeman, C. and Tobin, S. (1988) 'Enhancing the autonomy of mentally impaired nursing home resident. *The Gerontologist* 28, Supplement, 71–75.

Holland, T., Konick, A., Buffum, W., Smith, M. and Petchers, M. (1981) 'Institutional Structure and Resident Outcomes'. *Journal of Health and Social Behaviour* 22, 433–444.

Hughes, B. and Wilkin, D. (1980) *Residential Care of the Elderly: A Review of the Literature,* Research Report. Psychogeriatric Unit: University Hospital of South Manchester.

Kahana, E., Liang, J., Felton, B. (1980) 'Alternative models of person-environment fit: prediction of morale in three homes for the aged'. *Journal of Gerontology* 33 (4) 584–595.

Kimbell, A., Townsend, J. and Bird, M. (1974) *Elderly persons homes; a study of various aspects of regime and activities in elderly persons homes and their effect upon residents.* Mimeograph. Social Services Department, Cheshire.

King, R., Raynes, N., Tizard, J. (1971) *Patterns of Residential Care.* London: Routledge and Kegan Paul.

Kleemier, R. (1961) 'The use and meaning of time in special setting'. In Kleemier, R. (ed) *Aging and Leisure.* New York: Oxford University Press.

Lawton, M. (1974) 'Psychology of aging' In Brier W. (ed) *Aging: its challenge to the individual and society.* New York: Fordham University Press.

Lawton, M. (1979) *Environmental change: the older person as imitator and responder.* Mimeograph. Philadelphia: Philadelphia Geriatric Centre.

Lawton, M. (1982) 'Competence, environmental press and the adaptation of older people' In Lawton, M. Windley, P. and Byerts T. (eds) *Aging and the Environment. Theoretical Approaches.* New York: Springer.

Lemke, S. and Moos, R. (1980) 'Assessing the institutional policies of sheltered care settings', *Journal of Gerontology* 35 (1) 96–107.

Lemke, S. and Moos, R. (1981) 'The supra-personal environments of sheltered care settings'. *Journal of Gerontology* 36 (2) 233–43.

Moos, R. (1976) *The human context: environmental determinants of behaviour.* New York: John Wiley.

Moos, R. and Igra, A. (1980) 'Determinants of the Social Environments of Sheltered Care Settings'. *Journal of Health and Social Behavior* 21 (March), 88–98.

Moos, R.H. and Lemke, S. (1984) *Multiphasic Environmental Assessment Procedure (MEAP) Manual.* Social Ecology Laboratory, Stanford University, Palo Alto, California.

Moos, R. and Lemke, S. (1985) 'Specialised living environments for older people' In Birren, J. and Schaie, K. (eds) *Handbook of the psychology of aging.* New York: Van Nostrand Reinhold.

Norman, A. (1987) *Severe Dementia, the provision of long stay care, Report No. 7.* London: Centre for Policy on Ageing.

Pattie, A. and Gilliard, C. (1979) *Manual of the Clifton Assessment Procedures for Elderly (CAPE).* Sevenoaks: Hodder and Stoughton.

Pincus, A. (1968) 'The definition and measurement of the institutional environment in homes for the aged'. *The Gerontologist* 8 (3) 207–10.

Pincus, A. and Wood, V. (1970) 'Methodological issues in measuring the environment in institutions for the aged and its impact on residents', *International Journal of Ageing and Human Development* 1, 117–20.

Rabins, P. V., Merchant, A. and Nestadt, G. (1984) 'Criteria for diagnosing reversible dementia caused by depression: validation by 2 year follow up'. *British Journal of Psychiatry* 144, (5/84) 488–492.

Ransen, D. (1981) 'Long term effects of two interventions with the aged: an ecological analysis'. *Journal of Applied Developmental Psychology,* Spring 2 (1) 13–27.

Townsend, P. (1962) *The Last Refuge.* London: Routledge and Kegan Paul.

Wagner, G. (1988) *Residential Care, a Positive Choice: report of the Independent Review of Residential Care.* London: National Institute of Social Work, HMSO.

Willcocks, D., Peace, S. and Kellaher, L. (1987) *Private Lives in Public Places.* London: Tavistock.

Woods, R. and Britton, P. (1985) *Clinical Psychology with the Elderly.* London: Croom Helm Ltd.

CHAPTER 14

Resources, Needs and Outcomes in Community Services
Why Academic Caution Is Useful

Bleddyn Davies

'There is nothing more difficult to take in hand, more perilous to conduct, more uncertain in its success than to take the lead in the introduction of a new order of things' (Machiavelli).

Introduction

These are heady times in British community care. Since 1988, the British policy community has been bombarded with new ideas which amount almost to a new system of thought. Working through its principles has given a new clarity of purpose and a new confidence to parts of the British central administration. The pace of development of ideas is fast. The Department of Health (DOH) produces a steady stream of implementation guidance. Publications are appearing almost more quickly than they can be traced, far less read. Much good argument looks outdated by the time it is published, as researchers and commentators increasingly risk getting trapped into the time warp of their data collection.

Many local policy-makers too are genuinely excited by the new ideas. But their grasp of at least some of the new ideas is uneven. Some have traded steady development for quick returns, and have produced systems which are seriously flawed. (Indeed, some big noisy bangs have been quickly followed by what seems to have been ignominious and damaging busts.) Others are hastening slowly. Others are (as far as possible) avoiding the implementation of some disliked features of the policy, attempting to ignore or sidestep sanctions imposed by the centre.

So, implementation is uneven. As Sir Robin Butler (1990) commented about Machiavelli: 'Of course, he had only to deal with a whole lot of ambitious, scheming and murderous Italian princelings'. Sir William Pile's analogy between the central implementation of policies by local authorities and steering the Torrey Canyon[1] was a characteristically English understatement. More accurate would be the image of controlling a large fleet of Torrey Canyons through dark stormy nights, many steered by distracted officers constantly told what to do by mutinous committees of inexperienced and instantly dismissible crew.

National and local policy-makers will have to be entirely realistic about the scale and nature of the challenge if the policy is to succeed. For that reason they require periodic doses of purgative research evidence. This chapter uses some in an attempt to define the challenge more clearly.

Diversion From Residential Care: A Key End

White papers are the definitive statements of the policies which are reflected in government-sponsored legislation. The White Paper, Caring for People: Community Care in the Next Decade and Beyond, Cm 849 (1989), makes it clear that the diversion from residential modes of care is a central aim of the new policy. It is also assumed to be a crucial means. So a fair (if incomplete) test of the success of the policy will be whether it will reduce the proportion of spending on residential modes by increasing the expenditure on community-based care without greatly increased expenditure from public funds and worsening welfare outcomes, equity in the distribution of effort, and efficiency in public spending.

Begged Questions and Research Evidence: New Managerialist Argument

The New Managerialist Foci: Are They Too Narrow?

The evidence-based discussion of the nature and magnitude of the task consists mainly of what I have called the 'new managerialist' critique of community-based care and related literatures produced by academics. The new managerialist critique above all asserts that the principal challenge is to target resources better: to allocate publicly-financed resources to those whose care needs are greatest, who are at most risk of admission to institutions for long-term care, and who require their care to be financed by public expenditure; and so to allocate resources between recipients as to have the best effect on outcomes.

I argue that the new managerialist critique has underestimated the importance of some aspects of the causes and nature of the challenge. It has overstated the importance of targeting resources and underestimated challenges to the content and style of services because additional resource inputs seem usually to fail to have large impacts on important outcomes: challenges about the interplay of the ends and means and how they are perceived, the priorities and skills; and the investments in persons and structures. The influence of the new critique is powerful in most local agencies – indeed, there seem to be powerful levels of management in some social service departments (SSDs) at which it seems to be almost the main source of inspiration about the changes required. Used crudely, and not balanced by the kinds of imagination, sympathies and understanding brought by the best field professionals, there is often a danger that local policy argument will be mechanistic and, therefore, simplistic about some of the most difficult issues, and will be imprecise about the way the practice of managerial and field skills should be changed to achieve the required outcomes. This, I suspect, is a major threat to the success of a policy which has so much to commend it: not least, a clarity of logic and a new determination to manage change effectively than has been seen before in the history of community care.

The New Managerialist Foci and the Evidence

Let us take each of the aspects of targeting emphasized by the new managerialists in turn: first, vertical target efficiency: the proportion of resources used by persons not in high priority need; and second, matching levels of input to degrees of need.

Vertical Target Efficiency. Estimates of vertical target efficiency applying quite stringent criteria by the behavioral standards of the early 1980s suggested that vertical efficiency was high (Davies, Bebbington, Charnley and Colleagues 1990, p.17–18). It is more likely that measurement errors would have led to under, rather than over-estimation. However, the new policy suggests different targeting criteria. For instance, the targeting criteria implicit in the new policy would take more account of eligibility for means-tested services and the risk of inappropriate admission to residential care modes. So one cannot argue the importance of vertical target inefficiency on the basis of evidence analysed by the old criteria.

Matching Inputs to Levels of Need. Most commonly argued was that:

- sufficient and appropriate community-based care was not provided as an alternative for many most at risk of unnecessary admission to residential facilities; and
- the provision of standard home care services would be unlikely to divert demand from residential modes, because the risks of admission to institutional facilities seemed to be low.

The system starts from an excessively equal distribution in relation to need around low weekly levels. However effective inputs may be in making unnecessary admission to institutions for long-term care, such low levels and small variation make diversion of demand unlikely, the new managerialists argued.

The new managerialists alleged that first, allocations vary idiosyncratically; and second, more could be spent on the community-based care of some individuals without making that community-based care more costly to public funds than the least expensive residential mode. Research suggests that the degree of idiosyncrasy has been exaggerated. It has broadly supported the argument that more could be spent on community-based support for some, but – as we shall see later – it has changed our perception about how to correct the imbalance.

Equity, bias and consistency have been investigated by estimating degrees of equity, consistency and bias in targeting patterns. There is a clear distinction between 'equity' and 'consistency'. By equity, I mean allocations which are both consistent between persons in similar circumstances, and whose variations precisely reject criteria based on valid judgments about the values of costs and benefits. So equitable allocations are not biased in favour of some and against others. And allocations may be consistent without being equitable.

The findings suggest a degree of consistency similar to that found for similar services in Californian counties by Miller and Pruger before the agencies set about the task of increasing consistency (Pruger 1987). Allocations were most consistent within and between areas for recipients living alone; the traditional recipients of British home care. The evidence did suggest both bias and systematic differences in the prioritization between local governments. An example was the pattern of variation in allocations which would support informal carers (Davies *et al* 1990). The Californians certainly increased the consistency of allocations substantially (Davies *et al* 1990, p.229.) However, one surmises that it would be difficult to increase equity (by our definition) to the same degree because the removal of bias will require changed criteria by field allocators and expectations of those influencing patterns of demand.

The evidence likewise confirms the existence of a gap between the total per diem costs of what all but a very low proportion of recipients receive and the opportunity costs to public authorities of the least expensive mode of residential care. Figure 14.1 illustrates this for each of five groups. (The definitions of the groups are given in Table 14.3 below.) The information on which the figure is based does not allow an exact comparison of residential and community-based expenditures. Therefore, the figure systematically overstates the true gap between the costs of community-based and residential care. However, guesstimates of the size of the missing elements suggest that there remains a large difference between the effective maximum spending on community-based care and the opportunity costs of residential care. The best allocation would allow (but not automatically cause) publicly-financed community-based spending up to the level of the opportunity cost to the public authorities in the next more expensive residential mode of care, as long as admission to residential care would otherwise be certain and the two modes of care yielded equivalent welfare outcomes to dependants and significant others.

Complex and very local area variations (Davies, Darton and Goddard 1987) in the supply curves for services and other inputs suggest that what amounts to local shadow prices for services may lead to more equitable and efficient outcomes than attempts by agency policy-makers precisely to define the circumstances in which care should be provided in one mode rather than another (Davies *et al* 1990). Certainly discussions with leaders of case management agencies suggest vast variations in the position and slope of supply curves for alternative modes of care in the State of New York. Weissert, Cready and Pawelak (1988) reach a similar conclusion about the potential of shadow prices with the concentration and pooling of funds in the hands of case managers, though by another route.

The Social Services Inspectorate of the Department of Health has defined 'Cover' (the proportion of those potentially in need) and 'Intensity' (the average value of resources consumed by each recipient) to be crucial performance indicators. Their process analysis describes why and how the British system of the late-1980s was biased towards Cover at the expense of an effective and efficient level of Intensity, just as others did in the systems of the mid-1960s, using the same indicators (Davies 1968, Davies *et al* 1971).

The diagrams show (i) the average opportunity cost of care per week to the ssd for recipients living at home during the first six months (SSCOST), and (ii) average opportunity costs per week to the ssd and the community health services for people living at home during the first six months (SSHSCOST), (iii) the range of opportunity costs to the social service department of care for persons of that level of dependency in local authority old people's homes with the dependency needs found in 1981 (Homes, actual dependency mix), (iv) the range of opportunity costs for persons of that level of dependency in new local authority old people's homes, and (v) the sum of agency and opportunity costs to informal carers for persons of very high levels of dependency. Classification into group is by the circumstances of the most dependent client in the household. Frequencies are proportional to the area under the line.

The lines indicating the range of opportunity costs of places in local authority homes are from Davies and Goddard (1987). The opportunity costs to informal carers are estimated using the techniques described in *Community Services and the Social Production of Welfare* (PSSRU, 1991).

A. Long interval need, lesser informal support (Type 2)

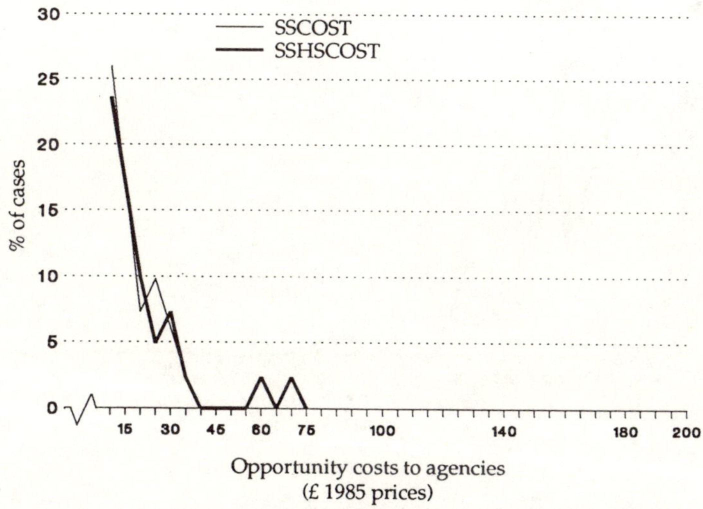

Figure 14.1: Community services and residential care costs

B. Short interval need, greater informal support (Type 3)

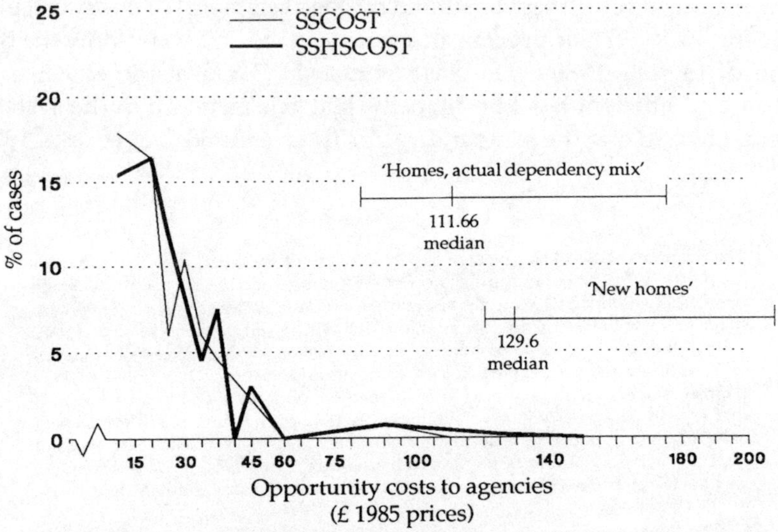

C. Short interval need, lesser informal support (Type 4)

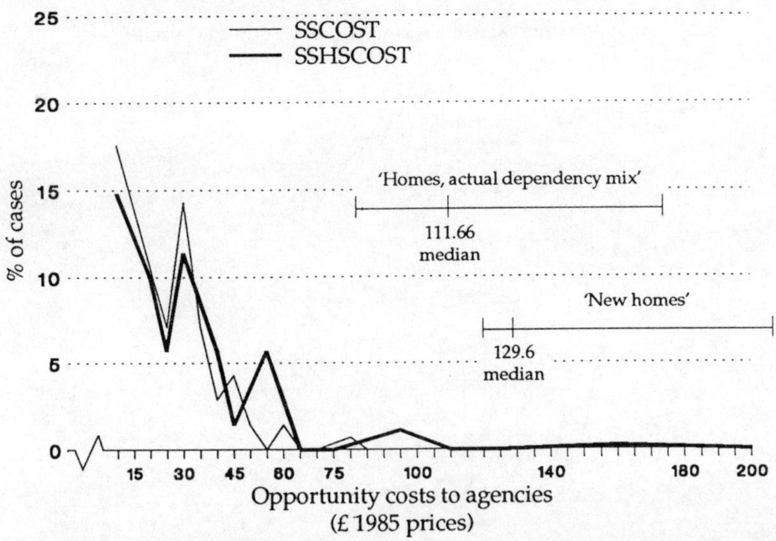

Figure 14.1: Community services and residential care costs (continued)

D. Critical interval need, greater informal support (Type 5)

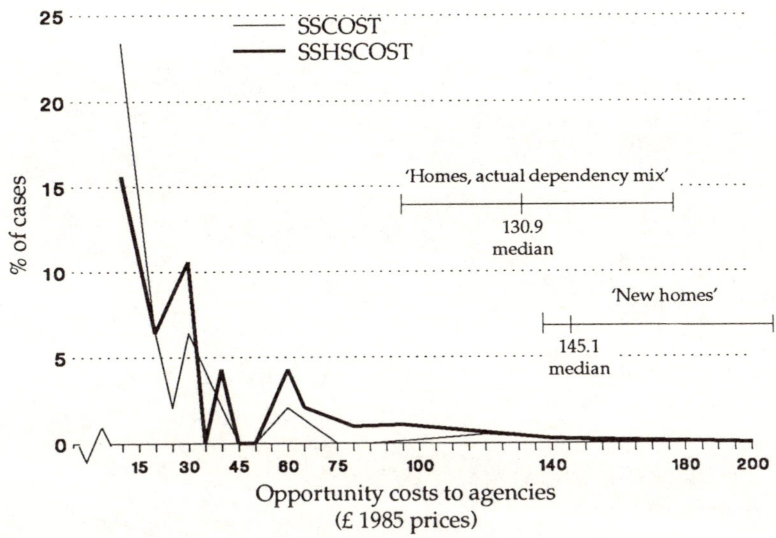

E. Critical interval need, lesser informal support (Type 6)

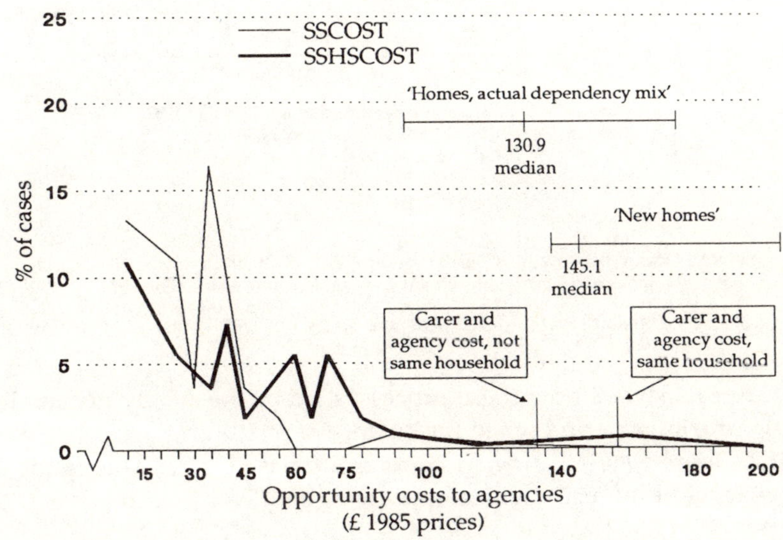

Figure 14.1: Community services and residential care costs (continued)

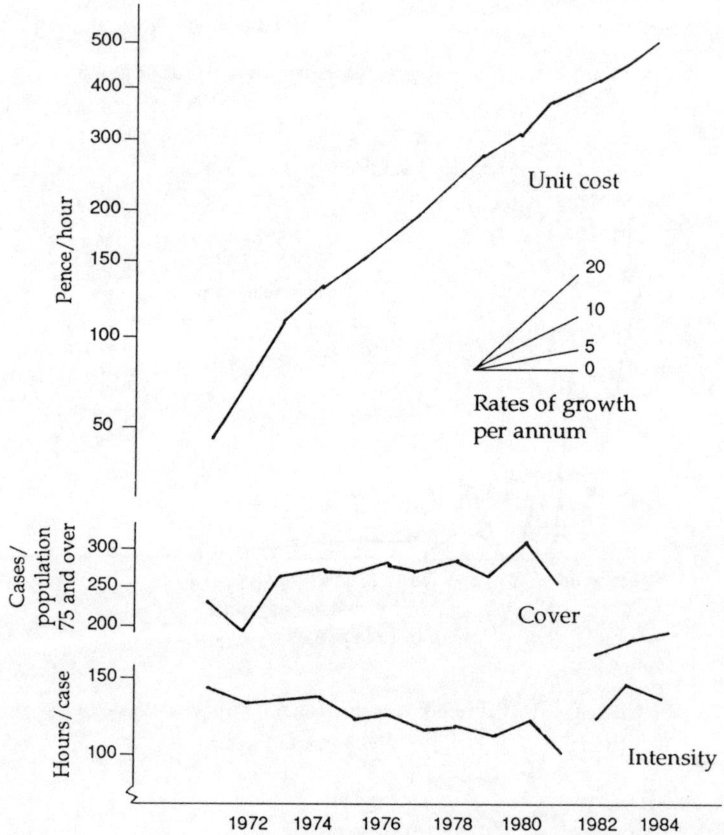

Note: Statistical discontinuity between 1981 and 1982
Sources: *Health and Personal Social Services Statistics*
Health Statistics for Wales
CIPFA: *Social Services Statistics: Actuals*
Population Trends

Source: Davies, Bebbington, Charnley and colleagues (1990) Resouces, Needs and Outcomes in Community-Based Care, Avebury/Gower, Aldershot

Figure 14.2: Cover, intensity and unit cost: England and Wales 1971–1984

Figure 14.2 shows how these processes led to the steady decline in the Intensity during a period when the balance of needs and publicly-financed resources were deteriorating in community-based care. The result is an average level of Intensity which appears to be lower than in several other countries, as is illustrated in Table 14.1.

Table 14.1 Intensity and cover in France, Scandanavia and England and Wales

	Cover: Cases/Population 65 and over	*Intensity: Hours per week*
France		
Haute Normandie, 1979–81	4.3[a]	5.0
Lille, 1979–81	8.3[a]	4.7
Ile de France, 1979–81, 1979–81	5.1	5.0
France, 1984	2.6	
Scandinavia		
Denmark	20[b]	4.9
Finland	10[b]	3.4
Norway	14[b]	3.3
Sweden	14[b]	6.8
England and Wales		
1985	6.0	2.6[c]
1986	6.1	2.4[c]
1988	4.6	3.2

Sources Ankri, J., Isnard, M.C. and Henrard, J.C. (1989); Brethouwer (1989); CIPFA (1987b, 1987b, 1990); Curtis and Bucquet (1987); Jansson and Wallberg (1988).
a In France home help is received only by those of low income.
b Proportion of elderly in households receiving home help.
c Hours received.

Source: Davies, Bebbington, Charnley and colleagues (1990) Resources, Needs and Outcomes in Community-Based Care, PSSRU Studies, Avebury/Gower, Aldershot.

Begged Questions: The Underrated Issues

New managerialist argument focuses primarily on resources; broadly conceived service categories, broad inputs, and money values. That the implications of other forms of argument must be worked through to these terms is undeniable. But so many of the challenges of community care can be related to resources only at the end of an argument worked out at another level and in different terms.

Some of these issues are: first, who exactly should be in the high priority target groups; second, the effects of higher levels of community-based services on circumstances which make necessary otherwise inappropriate admission to residential care; and third, the weight placed on costs criteria in case management and the influence exercised by case managers and others on the choice between residential and other care modes.

Let us discuss them in turn.

Who Should Have the Highest Priority?

Responsiveness to marginal productivities. The formal and general theoretical answer would be: those with whom the application of resources would yield the greatest ratio of the value of benefits to costs. This answer just begs the questions of real interest: what costs and benefits to whom? and how valued? But it does imply that other things being equal, those for whom service inputs yield the most beneficial change in outcomes overall should be within the target groups. That is, the high priority target groups should consist of types of case for whom there are likely to be high 'marginal productivities' of services for outcomes of ultimate evaluative significance.

There is surprisingly little American modelling of the relations between resources and outcomes or of targeting. Neither am I familiar with such modelling for countries other than the UK. However, Davies *et al* (1990) failed to find substantial and systematic responsiveness of who is a publicly-financed consumer of services to the predicted marginal productivities of services for them. Neither did the study find substantial and systematic responsiveness of the quantities consumed to the predicted marginal service productivities (Davies *et al* 1990, p.262–268). The marginal productivities investigated included both outcomes of ultimate evaluative significance for dependants and those for carers.

Convenient Over-Reductionism to Physical Disability. During the whole of the post-war period, British local governments have been slowly changing from being the providers of prescribed services to policy-making bodies for their areas (Stewart 1974; Committee on Management in Local Government 1967; Royal Commission on Local Government 1969). The progress has been halting and the goals confused (Stewart and Stoker 1988). It is a feature of this that social services departments have only recently begun to set targeting policies which define the priorities to be given to persons according to their circumstances, and even now, few have attempted it.

In the UK, as in some other places, senior managers tend to identify needs with incapacity to perform activities of daily living (ADLs) without help. This affects allocations in several ways.

1. Authorities are applying formulae which overstate the importance of physical disability in need judgements. It is a short step to embodying them in targeting criteria set by SSD headquarters and subsequently enforced by monitoring. We have seen such criteria set out, and have encountered authorities contemplating a move which could actually jeopardize the improvements in the equity and efficiency of allocations required, like the LIER system in the Netherlands or the late-lamented DMS scoring system in the State of New York. There is abundant evidence about the effects of using them. Field personnel tend first to make a judgement about the level of need, and then to complete their schedules in a way which yields a score which matches their prior judgement (Davies and Challis 1986, p.86, 105, 113; Davies *et al* 1990, p.296).
2. The Audit Commission (1985) provided a crude methodology for estimating local levels of need which is used by authorities for

> internal allocations. However, it relies excessively on physical disability. The methodology assumes constancy across areas in the proportions at different levels of physical disability with less informal support than would be needed to manage without social care, save for an adjustment for the proportion of elderly persons living alone. (The Audit Commission 1985, p.77, itself suggests that there are substantial area variations in the likelihood of support even at the regional level, and more variation at the local level.) Living alone is to be interpreted in a context set by many aspects of the physical and social environment.

Physical disability is only one cause of handicap. Cognitive impairment and the behavioural disturbance associated with it are, of course, correlated with physical disability but not to the degree to which only the latter need be estimated. Spector (1991) assessed the effects on estimates of adding moderate or severe cognitive impairment and disruptive behaviour to common American eligibility requirements based on functional disability criteria. The argument is that ADL questions typically ask about what cannot be done without assistance, and that persons with dementias are often not limited by physical disabilities, but either require supervision, prompting and cueing, or suffer behavioural disturbances which may jeopardize safety. He showed that the number of persons eligible for service was sensitive to criteria combining cognitive and disruptive behaviour with functional disability in various ways.

In some circumstances, the costs of resources can be used as the numeraire of need indicators, as the theoretical argument of the 1970s showed (Davies 1977). One cannot argue that the processes by which lifetime costs of social care have been determined were such that one could take them as indicators of the relative needs of clients and their informal carers. However, it would be surprising if the need-related circumstances which influenced them were completely unrelated to those influencing need judgments. So the features of statistical models which best predict lifetime costs of home and residential modes of long-term care would suggest what kinds of circumstance might predict lifetime needs.

Table 14.2 shows the equations predicting some (crude – indeed merely suggestive) estimates of lifetime costs subsequent to the sixth month of receipt of community-based service (Davies and Baines 1991a). What is interesting about them is that ADLs themselves far from dominate the equations. Features of the physical environment directly affect lifetime costs. So does cognitive impairment. Indirectly cognitive impairment and behavioural disturbance affect costs through their effects on carers, it seems. But relationships between the elderly persons and their informal carers are a leitmotif of the equations: for instance, whether or not the dependant has a confiding relationship, the nature of the declared motivation of principal informal carers. Indeed the equations remind us that it takes two to tango: the informal carers are not homogeneously reacting to the same dependent characteristics but bring their heterogeneous selves to the determination of the consumption of care, even in a system of publicly-financed care which is as insensitive to carer needs as the British social services of the 1980s.

Table 14.2 Prediction of costs at six month review: Equations for recipient groups.

	Costs To SSD	
	Home care	*Total Care*
Women Living Alone (87 cases)		
Area Price Level[2]	354.0**	0.179
Whether Central Heating	-523.8*	
Meals ADL Ability	-349.5****	0.472***
Housework ADL Ability		0.758**
Confused	-876.3***	
Critical Interval Need with Lesser Support		1.059**
Carer Sometimes angry with EP	-851.4***	
Carer Malaise Score		0.075*
Carer Reason for Caring is Duty	564.9*	
Carer has Long-standing Illness or Disability	550.2**	
Meals ADL Ability with Confidante		-0.747***
Personal Care ADL Ability with Confidante		0.748***
Housework ADL Ability with Personal Care ADL		-0.162**
Constant	*1505.5**	*4.432****
Adjusted R^2	*0.29****	*0.13**
Only Client in Household Is Male (33 cases)		
Area Price Level[2]	181.7	0.146
Personal Care ADL Ability	151.5**	-0.460****
Meals ADL Ability		0.557***
Some Incontinence	742.9**	0.349
Short Interval Need with Greater Support	1.359***	
Carer Reason for Caring is Love	-882.1**	
Carer Reason for Caring is Duty		-0.713
Carer Sometimes Angry with EP	-606.3*	
Some Incontinence with Carer Long Illness	1.102**	
Constant	*992.1*	*5.884****
Adjusted R^2	*0.38****	*0.54*****

Two Clients (Couple) in Household (37 cases)		
Area Price Level[2]	965.9****	0.493*
Either/both is/are Confused	-712.7**	
Meals ADL Ability	0.662****	
Serious Illness during Previous Six Months	-1.742****	
Carer has Good Relationship with EP(s)	1.664****	
Carer has Long-standing Illness or Disability	-2.083****	
Housework ADL among those with Central Heating	-0.128**	
Personal Care ADL Ability with Incontinence	0.276*	
Personal Care ADL with Reason for Caring is Duty	0.342**	
Constant	-2007.7**	4.645***
Adjusted R^2	0.36***	0.42****

Source: 1 Logarithmic transformation
2 One-tailed test
* Significantly different from (or if 2, greater than) 0 at 10% level
** Significantly different from (or if 2, greater than) 0 at 5% level
*** Significantly different from (or if 2, greater than) 0 at 1% level
**** Significantly different from (or if 2, greater than) 0 at 0.1% level

Other analyses show the complex interdependence of physical disability, cognitive impairment, and the nature and extent of the informal support. One example is a discriminant analysis predicting the admission of new community-based case clients to residential care during the subsequent six months (Davies *et al* 1990, p.86–92). So is the logit analysis of the probability of admission to institutions over 2.5 years (Davies and Baines 1991b). That analysis too reminds us of the way in which disability in general, and the particular form of the disability, work with other circumstances in a variety of ways to determine probabilities. It too reminds us that it takes two to tango. For instance, the analysis for women recipients living alone suggests that the presence of a confiding relationship is most influential when the circumstances of that relationship causes the kind of stress in which carers declare feelings of anger towards their dependants. Indeed, in this dance, there is important footwork between dependant, informal carer and a third group, the formal providers; although this is often not reflected in contact between agency and carer or in the conscious responsiveness of the agency to the carer's circumstances. An example from these models is that satisfaction with the nature of services seems to be a most important influence on lifetime costs of home care when taken in conjunction with the existence of someone described by the dependant to play the role of principal informal carer.

These equations are unusual only because they are based on a more extensive list of variables than is available for many predictions of utilisation.

The large number of variables allows the statistical models better to reflect the complexity.

Are those of high need also at high risk of admission to residential modes of care? The importance of the question is obvious. The substitution of community-based care for residential-based modes depends on concentrating the increased levels of community-based resources on a group whose members on average are likely to be admitted to residential-based modes if they are given only lower levels.

American experiments to substitute community-based for nursing home care illustrate the point. For whatever reason, the designers, managers and evaluators of these experiments did not make clear the difference between the two types of case, so the schemes usually appeared to fail by what was the one criterion used: whether they reduced public costs of care in institutions enough to compensate for the additional cost of community-based services and case managements. They failed to target those truly at high risk of institutional care.

The policy aims of the British White Paper suggest the same test as dominated American argument: whether the additional spending on community-based care will be compensated by reductions in spending on residentially-based modes. How important to success, by that criterion, will be the distinction between targeting at a population in high need and targeting at the population at high risk of admission to institutions for long-term care?

A Director's Dilemma. The importance of the question is obvious. Change must be made with little additional public spending. So it is important for better performance of case management tasks and the other content of the policy to allow substantial proportions now admitted to institutions for long-term care to be maintained at home at less cost to the SSD (DHSS 1987). However, that could only be achieved for many at high risk by providing a more appropriate service in quantity and nature. The Audit Commission (1985) and others were anyhow sceptical about the cost-effectiveness of using the provision of standard home care services to prevent unwanted and inappropriate admission, because the risks of admission among clients seemed, on average, to be low.

But, it has been argued that while the costs of concentration are clear, the effect on the proportion of persons needing residential modes is uncertain (Dexter and Harbert 1983). One reason for this is that a high proportion (up to 50%) of those admitted to residential modes have not previously been consumers of community-based care (Avon 1980, Barnes 1980, Bradshaw and Gibbs 1988, Neill *et al*, 1988; Sinclair 1990).

Directors are still articulating the same basic dilemma but in quantitative terms. How many persons of low need and risk would it be necessary to deprive of service in order to divert a substantial proportion of those at high risk from residential modes without worsening welfare outcomes? Lacking precise data, directors' sums are purely hypothetical. What we present here

Table 14.3 The need typology and proportions entering residential-based care within 2.5 years

Need type	*Definition*	*Case illustration*	*Per cent of all cases (weighted)*	*type entering*
0	Independent. 15 per cent of cases. people independent with respect of the main domestic tasks necessary to maintain an acceptable degree of sustenance, warmth, cleanliness, security.		3.8	11.0
1	Long interval needs. With potential/actual support. 16 per cent of cases. People who are unable to perform one or more domestic tasks which requires to be undertaken occasionally (less often than daily), but who have potential	Mr L. is 70 and lives alone. He had a 'minor stroke last year and although he says he could do most domestic tasks if he had to, he finds going out and managing steps difficult. He is well supported by friends and is visited regularly by his daughter in whom he can confide.	19.4	9.5
2	Long interval needs. Lacks potential support. 10 per cent of cases. People who are unable to perform one or more domestic tasks which need to be undertaken occasionally (less often than daily), and who lack adequate potential help.	Mr M., aged 84, lives alone and has partial hearing. He is quite mobile and goes out walking every day. Although he can manage to get himself drinks and snacks, he has difficulty managing cleaning since he is not used to doing these tasks and cooking himself a main meal. He has been well-supported in the past by his daughter, but she has recently become ill and has had to go into hospital.	15.1	9.5
3	Short interval needs. With potential/actual support. 16 per cent of cases. People who are unable to perform one or more domestic tasks which require to be undertaken frequently (more often than daily) but who have potential help.	Mr N. is 71 and lives alone. He has failing eyesight and is diabetic. He finds bathing, dressing and getting in and out of bed difficult. He cannot easily get out to do shopping but he can do light cleaning tasks. He cannot cook a main meal or snacks but can make himself a cup of tea. He is well supported by his sister who cooks for him, and he also has friends whom he sees regularly.	16.9	19.8

4	Short interval needs. Lacks potential/actual support. 21% of cases. People who are unable to perform one or more domestic which need to be undertaken frequently (more often than daily) and who lack adequate potential help.	Mrs O. is aged 85 and lives alone in her own house of which she is very proud and does not want to leave. She is blind in one eye and suffers from leg ulcers which have to be dressed by a district nurse three times a week. She used to share her home with her son but he died suddenly last year. He used to do the shopping and lots of jobs around the house. Mrs O. no longer goes out now that her son cannot take her. She finds a number of domestic and self-care tasks very difficult, and some she cannot manage at all. Her niece visits her once a week and she sometimes asks the paper boy to run errands for her. She worries that she will not be able to continue coping living alone.	19.5	17.1
5	Critical interval needs. With potential/actual support. 11% of cases. People who are unable to perform crucial self-care tasks which need to be undertaken frequently and at short notice, but who have potential help.	Mr P. is aged 77 and lives with his wife aged 67. She is quite fit and able to take care of the domestic tasks in to the house and to care for herself. Mr P. had a stroke recently and was in hospital for some time. He is housebound and can do almost nothing for himself. A district nurse calls twice weekly to bath him, and he also receives physiotherapy. Mr and Mrs P. are closely involved with a local church community and friends/ volunteers call daily. These friends are available to sit with Mr P. while Mrs P. goes out, and to take them both out.	12.8	28.0
6	Critical interval needs. Lacks potential/actual support. 19 % of cases. People who are unable to perform crucial self-care tasks which need to be undertaken frequently and at short notice, and who lack adequate potential help.	Mr Q. is 78 and lives with his wife who is 80. He suffered a stroke some years ago and is confined to a wheelchair, having lost the use of his legs. Although Mrs Q. helps him in and out of bed, she has considerable difficulty herself in looking after the house. A district nurse calls to bath Mr Q. about once a month. Mr and Mrs Q. are rather isolated, having no contact with friends or relatives. Mr Q. worries about becoming too dependent to be cared for at home and is conscious of overburdening his wife.	12.6	22.6

is a model of the consequences of diversion targeted on broad need categories. It is 'lexicographic'. Diversion for members of the most promising category is exhausted before diversion of others is allowed, and the diversion is at the expense of the denial of service only of those in low need category. (Of course, the art of the case manager is to pick out the likely candidates across the board. But the statistical analysis required for that is not available to directors.)

Evidence for the late-1980s has been analysed by Davies *et al* (1990). The evidence is about need-related circumstances of new clients and their informal carers, changes in needs and costs over 2.5 years. (However, as we have argued, the results for marginal productivities should be treated as irrelevant to the quantification of the dilemma for the medium-run, since we argue that a main objective of policy should be to secure their great improvement.) Table 14.3 provides a simplified description of two types of evidence needed: numbers of clients at various levels of need, and average probabilities of admission to care.

Consider an authority whose targeting and costs were typical of the late-1980s. The director and his colleagues may start by considering the proportion of low need persons – Types 0, 1 and 2: 38% of the total – who would have to be deprived of service to finance an attainable diversion in a group at higher risk of residential admission – say Type 6, the group with the second highest probability. Davies and Baines (1991a) estimate the lifetime costs to the social services department of both home and residential care to be high: £1559 and £3916 respectively. (Type 5 clients, which have the highest probability of admission to institutions, have low expectations of life, a comparison of Figures 14.5a and 14.5b of *Resources Needs and Outcomes* suggest, and so are typically less good candidates for diversion.)

On average the weekly costs of the services they actually obtained is about £25 (Davies *et al* 1990, Table 3.14). The average allocation to Type 6 clients in the mid-1980s was low: for instance, 5 hours a week of home help, 4 meals, and 1 day care session among those who actually received these services (Davies *et al* 1990, Tables 3.2, 3.4 and 3.7). So the case managers could well believe that the unwanted admission of some at least of the Type 6 clients could be avoided with (say) a doubling of the resources on average to members of the group. (Ten hours of home care with meals daily and 2 sessions of day care would not seem unreasonable to achieve this with what is a very dependent group with hard-pressed carers.) That would raise the average for the group so targeted to £50 per week.

However, Table 14.3 also shows that the probability of this group actually entering residential care even over 2.5 years is only 0.23. Perhaps with the exercise of case managers' judgment, it could be halved. (One would not expect prospective predictions to be very good, since so many random events affect the likelihood of admission to institutions for long-term care: an unexpected health accident to a carer, an unexpected acceleration in decline in a period of unusually bad weather...) So the higher costs would

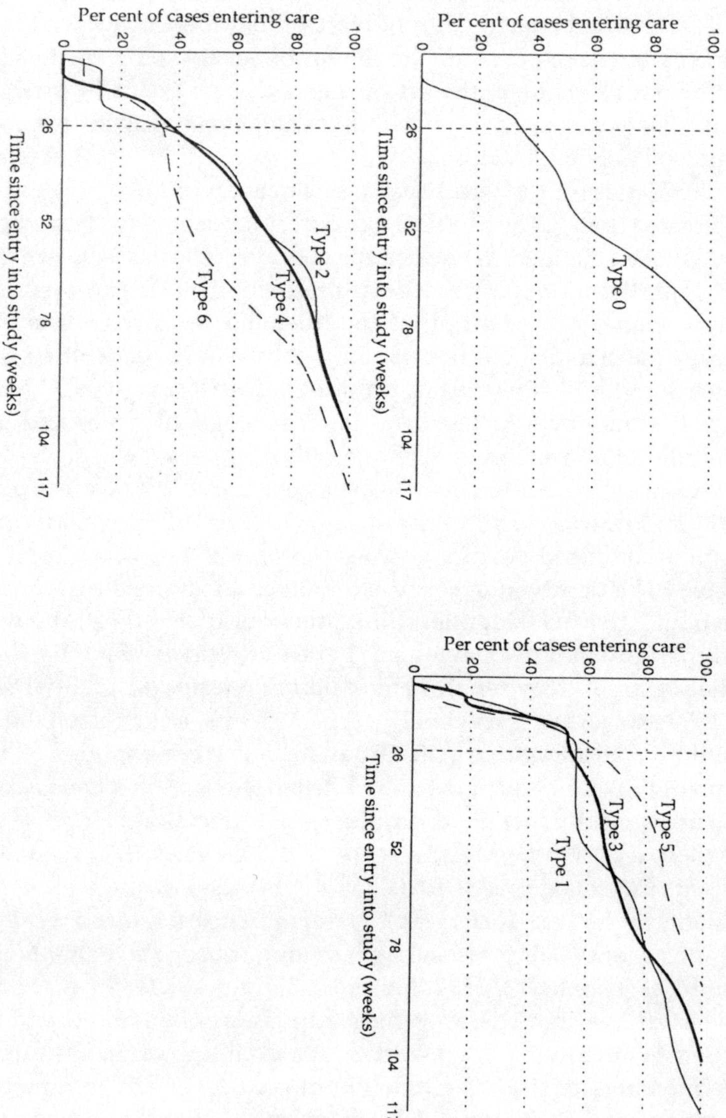

Figure 14.3: Timing of admission to residential care by need typology of client group

have to be borne for twice as many cases as would be diverted over the 2.5 years; £100 in all per case diverted. That would be £2(50)-25 = £75 more than the actual average expenditure on the Type 6 cases.

The most obvious offsetting saving is the reduction in the cost of residential care of Type 6 clients. The median cost in residential care for persons of equivalent dependency was then of the order of £130 weekly at the same 1984 price level (Davies *et al* 1990, Figure 1E). Figure 14.3 suggests that persons with Type 6 circumstances who enter residential care tend to be admitted later than most. Therefore the area under the curve is relatively small, and the average proportion of the time spent in residential care is relatively large; say 12 months (or less). This implies an average offsetting cost saving on residential care of 40% of the difference between residential and the new home care costs for each person who would otherwise been admitted; ie £0.4(130–100) = £12. So the net cost of diversion might be £63; £(75–12).

That must be compared with the costs of the 38% of low need clients in Types 0, 1 and 2. The weekly costs of these low need clients to the SSD was just over £10. (The lifetime costs to the SSD of home care and residential care for persons living alone and from Types 1 and 2 were estimated to be £1072 and £815 respectively; low compared with those for Type 5.)

Assume first that there are no effects of the removal of provision on the probability of admission to residential modes of the low need groups. Then the prevention of admission of one Type 6 client might require the denial of service to some 6.3 low need clients. Assume also that the total number of cases is 100; 38 in the low need groups and 13 in Type 6, the same distribution as in Table 2. Then the cost of diverting about one case in four would be the denial of service to 25 persons in the low need groups; 65% of all low need cases.

However, low need cases denied services might, as a result, have a higher probability of admission to residential care, partly because of their deterioration to join groups with higher probabilities. That would raise the cost of concentration. It would require only 1.7%, of the denied cases to spend an additional 12 months in homes (at the Figure 1B median cost of £112) to force the denial not only to the other low need cases also, but to some Type 3 and 4 cases (because the additional persons in the low need groups would also have enhanced probabilities of residential admission). That in turn would have greater knock-on effects on expected residential costs.

Type 6 is not the only group from which diversion would be considered. On the one hand, the cost of diversion of some of the cases would be reduced because of their lesser dependency and so lower cost requirements for diversion, but this is partly offset by their lower probabilities of entering homes and the longer average period before doing so resulting in lower savings on residential costs achieved by the diversion. There is substantial relative variation in the probabilities shown in Table 14.3.

However, whether the increased spending on community-based services would in fact reduce the need for residentially-based modes sufficiently will depend not only on who is being targeted, but also on the welfare outcomes of the additions to spending. Let us call the improvement in an outcome resulting from a unit increase in a service the 'marginal productivity' of that service. The proposition can then be rephrased: whether increased spending on community-based services for those in high need will depend not just on targeting, but also on the marginal productivities of services for crucial outcomes which determine whether welfare overall would be better in a community-based or on another care mode.

The Effects of Increased Inputs on Need-related Circumstances: 'Marginal Productivities'

The new managerialist critique did not suggest that marginal productivities of services alone or in combination was a major cause for anxiety, though there were particular criticisms (Audit Commission 1985, Social Services Inspectorate 1987). Neither did it comment on the symptoms of low marginal productivities: high marginal costs of outcomes – though at least some of the research literature had shown high marginal costs for recipients of conventional provision with exactly the characteristics which put them at high risk of inappropriate admission to institutions for long-term care (Challis and Davies 1986, Davies and Challis 1981, Davies and Challis 1986). Moreover, the channeling reports clearly suggested low productivities for nursing home utilization (Brown and Phillips 1986), though scrutiny of appendices to project reports on other outcomes suggests that they undertook nothing approximating the estimation of marginal productivities of service inputs for other outcomes.

So there has been little large-scale research to estimate marginal productivities. A study by colleagues and I of the British system suggests generally low marginal productivities for outcomes important for avoiding the need for residential care. They are low not just for outcomes whose importance is suggested by the literature about what factors influence admission to residential care, but also for outcomes whose definitions were tied closely to what front-line managers and workers saw to be the main aims of the service.

Table 14.4 illustrates the estimated effects of varying service levels on outcomes related to remaining in the community. The relationships are perverse. These perverse relationships reflect the fact that the beneficial effects of higher service levels were insufficient to drown the noise created by measurement and specification errors. (Brown and Phillips 1986 found the same phenomenon.) One should not be surprised that the link between service inputs and admission and residential care is weak. Front-line managers mentioned the prevention of admission in fewer than one case in five when asked the purposes of the proposed interventions. Likewise there were effects on dependants' morale score for only some types of case. (Again this was component with what front-line allocators described to the aims for the individual cases). As in most American studies, there were not general effects on functional capacities (Kemper 1988). The main shaft of light in the gloomy Dutch landscape was the effect on customers' view of the impact of the home help service. That is illustrated in the third column of the table. Redesigning models around the social production of welfare [SPOW] variant (Netten and Davies 1990; Qureshi, Challis and Davies 1988) of the Personal Social Services Research Unit's (PSSRU's) production of welfare approach produced a few other rays of light but did not greatly change the picture (PSSRU 1992, forthcoming).

Table 14.4 Predicted destinational outcome of a 'typical' Social Services client, given different levels of domiciliary services

Service	*Entered institution* %	*Died* %	*Social services enabled client to live at home* %	*Other survivors* %
No home help/no meals on wheels	3	4	5	88
2 hours home help/no meals on wheels	4	5	5	86
4 hours home help/ 2 meals on wheels p.w.	5	6	17	72
8 hours home help/5 meals on wheels p.w.	6	7	61	26
No social work	3	6	9	82
Low social work	3	6	10	81
Moderate social work	15	7	12	67
High social work	84	2	3	11
(N)	(40)	(34)	(84)	(324)

Note: Reading along rows, the above figures give the predicted probability of each destinational outcome, using the discriminant equations of Table 3.5. The predicted probabilities are calculated by taking every variable at its mean value, except the indicated service input.

Source: Davies, Bebbington, Charnley and colleagues (1990) Resources, Needs and Outcomes in Community-Based Care, PSSRU Studies, Aldershot: Avebury\Gower

So for outcomes for dependants, the investigation found that:

- few of the marginal productivities important for achieving the substitution of community-based for residential care modes were large enough to be heard through the noise;
- the marginal productivities for the harder outcomes could not be detected: the probability of admission to institutions for long-term care, the number of days spent consuming home care, the number spent in residential institutions receiving long-term care, indicators of the capacity to perform ADLs and the like;

- the softer outcomes may have been influenced more, but the results can be interpreted in various ways.

The results for outcomes for carers were equally disappointing. What is clear is the great stress which substantial proportions of carers face, not always solely caused but, judging from the correlation of stress and dependant characteristics, usually exacerbated by their caring activities. Figure 14.4

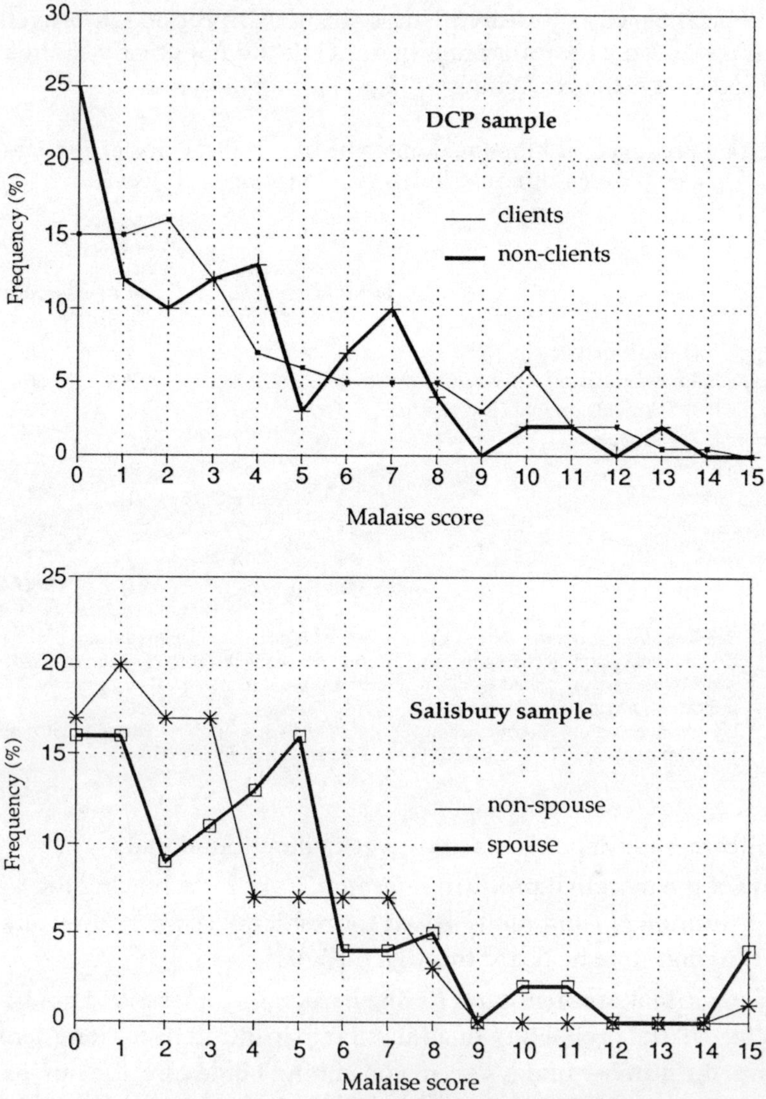

Notes: In the Domiciliary Care (DCP) sample,all principle carers were non-spouse.
Source: Davies, Bebbington, Charnley and colleagues (1990) Resources, Needs and Outcomes in Community-Based Care, PSSRU Studies, Avebury/Gower, Aldershot

Figure 14.4: Distribution of principle carers malaise scores

describes the distributions of principal informal carers by their score on the Rutter Malaise Inventory (Rutter, Tizard and Whitmore 1970). Rutter and his colleagues suggested that scores of 5 or 6 are outside the normal range and indicate stress (Quine and Pahl 1985). Our modelling suggested that inputs of the community-based services affected Carer Malaise for carers in only relatively rare circumstances (Davies *et al* 1990, p.266–268).

So it is as important to raise marginal productivities as it is simply to ensure that targeting policy consciously reflects the fact that high need cases are not necessarily at high risk of admission to institutions for long-term care.

Marginal productivities are about resource inputs. The statistical effects comparable to marginal productivities for non-resource inputs have been better studied than marginal productivities themselves. There is a good reason. The 'ologists – sociologists, gerontologists and psychologists – are of course right: the effects on outcomes of variations in the non-resource inputs which they study are more immediate and larger than those of resources inputs in the systems we study, though partly because the 'ologists have had more influence on service ideologies than have economists or system scientists. PSSRU work which simultaneously estimates the effect of resource and non-resource inputs confirms the greater influence of variations in non-resource inputs.

Case Management Tasks and Arrangements

The Relevance of Case Management Tasks.

Each of the main planks of the new policy for community care will affect targeting propensities, the marginal productivities of services, and the costs of achieving target outcomes for persons in different circumstances. However, the most directly influential is the recognition of the relationship between the performance of core tasks of case management and efficiency, and the arrangements made to secure that. How their performance affects efficiency aspects has been argued elsewhere (Davies and Challis 1986, p.20–24).

There are various reasons why the efficient performance of case management tasks affects productivities. The first is that case management involves the mixing of inputs to produce the outcomes, and the contribution to the outcomes of each additional building block depends on how, when and for whom that block is used. Second, some outcomes contribute more to welfare than do others, and case managers set out to influence the outcome mix so that it reflects relative valuations. Third, better performance of core tasks provides information about the nature of needs, so helping to guide the nature and content of the service provided. Fourth, better performance can create incentives to make services fit client needs better: if one service does not perform well, another can be used which produces some of the same outcomes. Note how the extent of these benefits reflect the precise arrangements for the performance of tasks; for instance, the scope of the tasks performed, the span of the resources commissioned and outcomes sought.

The Evidence About the Effectiveness of Case Management.

The PSSRU experiments have produced notable gains (Challis and Davies 1986, Challis *et al* 1989, Challis *et al* 1990, Chesterman, Challis and Davies 1991, Davies and Challis 1986). They were clearly successful by various criteria. The White Paper and other Department of Health (DH) documents referred to the authorities which had introduced arrangements based on the PSSRU experiments. Perhaps because of that, many seem to think that some of the features of PSSRU models should automatically be incorporated.

However, the results of PSSRU models are not a good guide to what might be expected from the better performance of case management tasks. They are not even a good guide to the results of models with their most characteristic features: concentration of responsibility, authority and accountability for performing most aspects of a wide range of core tasks on persons with delegated budgets, from which are met all the costs of resources commissioned for long-term care. The reason is that (like, for instance the North Carolina CCP), the PSSRU experiments were primarily based on secondary referral of persons for whom what they had to offer was expected to make admission to institutions unnecessary. They have operated with small caseloads and skilled personnel for clients for whom case-managed care was expected to be most beneficial; not a general selection of cases, or even a general selection of high need cases.

There are several reasons why the universal application of the PSSRU model to all clients would be impracticable, indeed inefficient. The most persuasive is that the arithmetic of resources would not add up.

For evidence about the effects of models with case managers but with larger caseloads we must turn to American experiments. A review of the costs and benefits based on project reports and meta-evaluations suggested that their gains were less than in the PSSRU experiments (Davies *et al* 1990, p.306–310). However, they also faced more handicaps than in similar models in British SSDs. The White Paper opted for what Kemper (1990) called 'a single agency system' for case management. In particular, the SSD, the exclusive gatekeeper for most members of the target subgroup financed most from public funds, and the agency also undertakes the associated systems activities: the development and implementation of the whole range of 'trade and industry' policies required in local mixed economies of care. The UK is starting from a collectivist and politically accountable monopoly, whereas the US is starting from a highly imperfect and fragmented market. The causes of its failures are hugely buttressed by powerful interest groups – so British outcomes should be better.

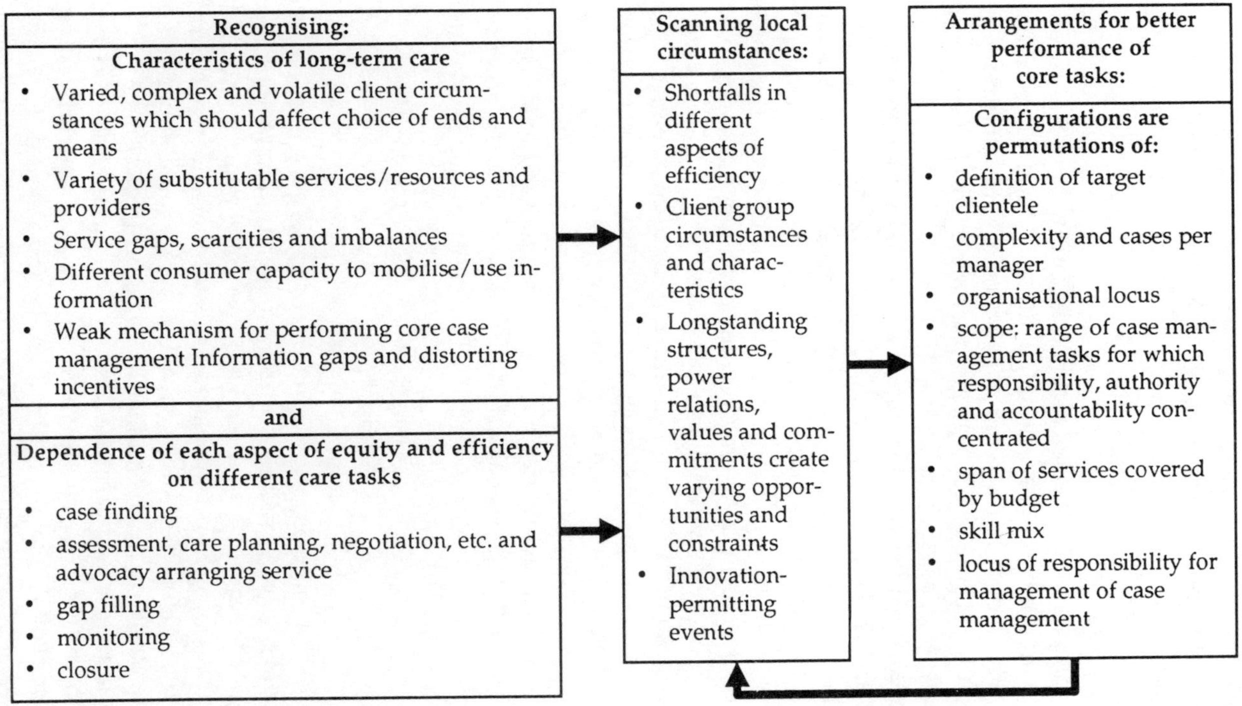

Source: Davies, Bebbington, Charnley and colleagues (1990) *Resources, Needs and Outcomes in Community-Based Care*, PSSRU Studies, Avebury/Gower, Aldershot

Figure 14.5: PSSRU Community care approach: managerial scanning to improve arrangements for performing core case management tasks

Fitting Case Management Arrangements To Client and System Characteristics.

The costs and benefits of alternative arrangements differ according to the characteristics of client type and system characteristics. The repertoire of ways of performing the core tasks is vast; formed from permutations of aspects of arrangements. Only some concentrate responsibility, authority and accountability for core case management tasks. Only some separate case management and commissioning from supply. They differ in the range of skills, inputs, caseloads, span of case management tasks, skill levels, and other important ways.

Some authorities which have acted most decisively in the introduction of case-managed community care have adopted models with clear and serious contradictions which put at risk some of the most important equity and efficiency gains which could be brought good arrangements for performing core case management tasks.

Because the costs and benefits of alternatives differ, and because the international literature is producing evidence which can help the matching of arrangements to circumstances, it is important to develop what we call a 'contingency theory of case management'. Its purpose is to develop an argument about what features of arrangements for achieving the performance of case management tasks are likely to be the most cost-effective in different contexts. By distinguishing several, indeed many features which distinguish arrangements, this approach shifts the focus to combinations of arrangements from the simplest typologies. That is important. Such simple typologies are too general to do more than introduce the policy-maker to the idea of variations in arrangements. They do not support argument of the sophistication needed for design decisions. Our first attempt which is more than a few pages in length is contained in *Resources Needs and Outcomes in Community-Based Care* (Davies *et al* 1990). The kinds of categories these discussed are illustrated in Figure 14.5.

Conclusions

1. There is a real risk of confusing two definitions of the target group: persons in high need and persons at risk of admissions to institutions for long-term care and eligible for means-tested services. Case management will not in itself cause such extensive and widespread substitution at low service cost as to finance the expansion of community-based care for all those in high need. Wishful thinking (and perhaps the desire of interest groups to promote community-based care) are likely to make this confusion more likely. The point has been made with increasing vociferousness by American analysts (Callahan 1989, Weissert, Cready and Pawelak 1988). One must promote better community-based care for those in substantial need and without the assets to pay for themselves because it is worth the public money in its own right.

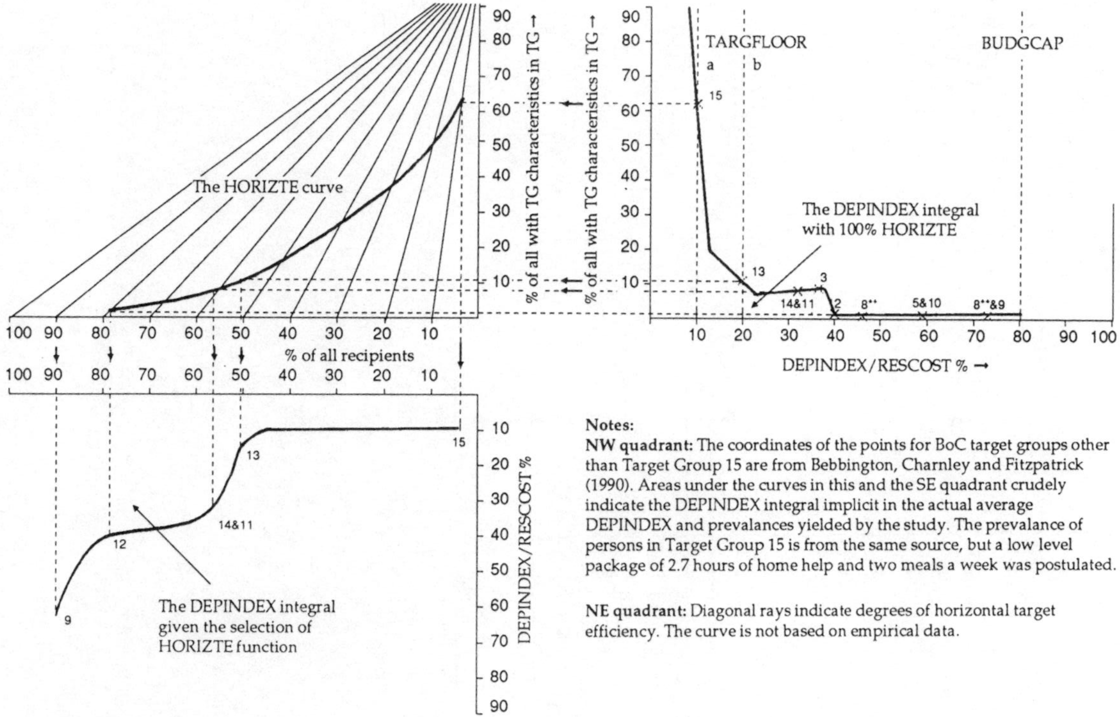

Notes:

NW quadrant: The coordinates of the points for BoC target groups other than Target Group 15 are from Bebbington, Charnley and Fitzpatrick (1990). Areas under the curves in this and the SE quadrant crudely indicate the DEPINDEX integral implicit in the actual average DEPINDEX and prevalances yielded by the study. The prevalance of persons in Target Group 15 is from the same source, but a low level package of 2.7 hours of home help and two meals a week was postulated.

NE quadrant: Diagonal rays indicate degrees of horizontal target efficiency. The curve is not based on empirical data.

Source: Davies, Bebbington, Charnley and colleagues (1990) *Resources, Needs and Outcomes in Community-Based Care*, PSSRU Studies, Avebury/Gower, Aldershot

Figure 14.6: DEPINDEX Distributions, Horizte Judgements, and the effects of varying Targfloor

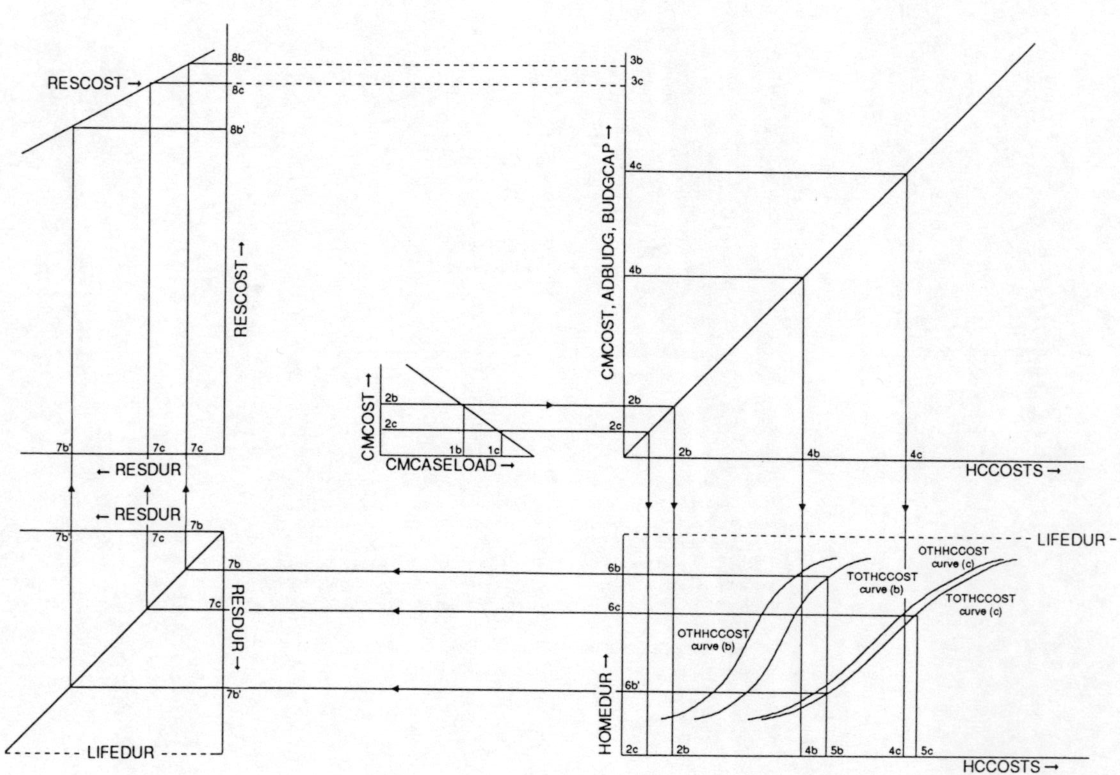

Source: Davies, Bebbington, Charnley and colleagues (1990) *Resources, Needs and Outcomes in Community-Based Care*, PSSRU Studies, Avebury/Gower, Aldershot

Figure 14.7: Cost relationships and case management parameters

2. Good targeting requires subtlety and sophistication. However, we are hopefully in transition from supply-led patterns through demand-led patterns to patterns which are more needs-led. Good trade and industry policy – for instance, the development of information for long-term planning by suppliers and others, the monitoring of policy performance – will become more not less necessary as we move towards that third phase. It is then that we shall need new descendants of earlier work on balance of care modelling and territorial justice studies.
3. We have always in fact varied the proportions in need actually receiving service – i.e. horizontal target efficiencies. However, the variation has been uncontrolled and unstudied; too much determined by arbitrary supply factors. There will always be a need to equate demand and financial resources. We should begin working on ways of squaring explicit decisions about priorities in the meeting of need – i.e. relative horizontal target efficiencies. Figure 14:6 illustrates what I have in mind.
4. It will be important to develop the contingency theory of case management. Some of that theory should focus on broad structural arrangements and the investments required for them. The scanning argument in Figure 14.5 illustrates the kinds of focus for that kind of argument. Other bits of theory should be about how to make the best use of resources by the frequent adjustment of some case management parameters. Take the argument of Figure 14.7. First we must explore what types of case management arrangements will yield what parameters for the S-shaped lines of the south-east quadrant. Then we must work simultaneously to fix horizontal target efficiencies, budget caps and average budgets, case management arrangements and the like so as to achieve an efficient allocation of resources. This is an argument designed for arrangements with devolved budgets financing the range of substitute inputs held by case managers.

As Kemper has recently argued, the research of the last decade did not engage the questions which we now face. The strengths and weaknesses of the collections were chosen with different perceptions of the issues in mind. This is a formidable agenda for us all.

However, there are ways of stretching public finance further which are not extensively considered in the British literature. One is to create insurance-related mechanisms to help users finance much of their own long-term social care. The Griffiths' Report took up some of the Matching concepts in a section about the long run, recommending studies of some of the models (Davies and Challis 1986, p.537–542; Griffiths 1988, paras 6.59–6.63). No doubt it is too politically sensitive to have been discussed in the White Paper (Griffiths 1988). However there are potentially important gains for public policy, as I illustrated in Davies (1986) and Davies and Challis (1986). The question is now not whether such mechanisms will emerge (some are well established already, and others are being introduced by the day) but whether they will be affordable by those who might potentially spend down their assets to become eligible for means-tested benefits if they were to spend a long time in long-term care need. We need to follow through the analyses which preceded and informed the discussion of public-private partnerships in the Pepper Report. In successive visits to the US during the last dozen years, I have watched the growth of such partnerships directed at achieving the goals of public policy. But that is another subject.

Notes

1. The supertanker Torrey Canyon ran aground on the Pollard Rock off the South West coast of England in 1967. The abandoned wreck released 30,000 tonnes of oil and contaminated 100 miles of Cornish beaches. The event provided the British media with its first major domestic 'pollution by oil-slick' story, and substantially raised levels of public awareness about the hazards of transporting oil by sea.

References

Ankri, J., Isnard, M. and Henrard, J. (1989) *Home help in France.* Paris: Laboratoire Santé et Vieillissement, Université René Descartes.

Audit Commission for England and Wales (1985) *Managing social services for the elderly more effectively.* London: HMSO.

Avon Social Services Departmnet (1980) *Admissions to homes for the elderly: A survey of alternatives.* Bristol: Avon County Council.

Barnes, C.D. (1980) *The relentless tide: A study of admission into homes for the elderly.* Kingston-upon-Thames: Surrey County Council.

Bebbington, A.C. and Davies, B.P. (1983) 'Equity and efficiency in the allocation of the personal social services'. *Journal of Social Policy* 12 (3) 309–330.

Bradshaw, J. and Gibbs, I. (1988) *Public support for private residential care.* Aldershot: Gower/Avebury.

Brethouwer, D. (1989). *Ongelijkles in het Geltrush van Eezinsvergorgy,* Doctoral Dissertation, University of Groningen, The Netherlands.

Brown, R., and Phillips, B. (1986) *The effects of case management and community services on the impaired elderly.* Princeton, NJ: Mathematica Policy Research.

Butler, Sir R. (1990) *Managing change: The Redcliffe-Maud Memorial Lecture 1990.* London: Royal Institute of Public Administration.

Callahan, J.J., (1989) 'Play it again Sam – there is no impact'. *The Gerontologist* 29, 5–6.

Capitman, J. (1985) *Evaluation of co-ordinated community orientated long-term care demonstration programs.* Berkeley, California: Berkeley Planning Associates.

Capitman, J. (1986) 'Community-based long-term care models, target groups and impacts on service use'. *The Gerontologist* 46, 389–397.

Caring for people: Community care in the next decade and beyond. Cm 849, London: HMSO (1989)

Challis, D., Chessum, R., Chesterman, J., Luckett, R., and Traske, K. (1990) *Case management in social and health care.* University of Kent at Canterbury, England: PSSRU.

Challis, D., Darton, R., Johnson, L., Stone, M., Traske, K., and Wall, B. (1989) *Supporting frail elderly people at home.* University of Kent at Canterbury, England: PSSRU.

Challis D. and Davies, B.P. (1986) *Case management in community care.* Aldershot: Gower.

Chartered Institute of Public Finance and Accountancy (1987) *Personal social services statistics, 1985–6: Actuals.* London: CIPFA.

Chartered Institute of Public Finance and Accountancy (1990) *Personal social services statistics, 1988–9: Actuals.* London: CIPFA.

Chesterman, J., Challis, D. and Davies, B.P. (1991) *Experimental evaluation of case-managed community care in routine programmes: Kent schemes of the mid-1980s.* Discussion Paper 773, University of Kent at Canterbury, England: PSSRU, .

Committee on the Management of Local Government (1967) *Management of local government I: Report of the Committee.* London: HMSO.

Cortis, S. and Bucquet, D. (1987) 'Characteristics of elderly people receiving home-help in three regions of France'. *Revue d'Epidemiologie et de le Santé Publique* 35, 318–322.

Davies, B.P. (1968) *Social Needs and Resources in Local Services.* London: Joseph.

Davies, B.P. (1977) 'Need and outputs'. In Heisler, H. (ed) *Foundations of social administration.* Basingstoke: Macmillan.

Davies, B.P. (1986) 'American lessons for British public policy research on long-term care of the elderly.' *Quarterly Journal of Social Affairs* 2, 321–344.

Davies, B.P. (1987) 'Equity and efficiency in community care: supply and financing in an age of fiscal austerity'. *Ageing and Society* 7, part 2, 129–162 and 237–240.

Davies, B.P. (1988) 'Making a reality of community care: A critique of the Audit Commission Report'. In Davies, B.P. and Knapp, M. (eds) 'The production of welfare approach: Some new PSSRU argument and results'. *British Journal of Social Work Supplement* 18, 173–188.

Davies, B.P. (1990) 'New priorities in home care: Principles from the PSSRU experiments'. In Howe, A. Ozanne, E. and Selby Smith, C. *Community care policy and practice: New directions in Australia.* Melbourne: University of Monash Press, 47–72.

Davies, B.P. and Baines, B. (1991a) *On lifetime costs and targeting: Effects of current case management policy on future resource commitments with entropic assumptions about productivities.* Discussion paper 738, University of Kent at Canterbury, England: PSSRU.

Davies, B.P. and Baines, B. (1991b) *On the determinants of the probability of admission to residential institutions for long-term care among new recipients of community-based services.* Discussion Paper 774. University of Kent at Canterbury, England: PSSRU.

Davies, B.P., Barton, A.J., Macmillan, I.S., and Williamson, V.K. (1971) *Variations in services for the aged: A causal analysis.* London: Bell.

Davies, B.P., Bebbington, A.C., Charnley, H., and Colleagues (1990) *Resources, needs and outcomes in community-based care: A comparative study of the production of welfare in ten local authorities in England and Wales.* Avebury, Aldershot: PSSRU Studies.

Davies, B.P. and Challis, D. (1981) *The Thanet Community Care Project: Some interim results.* Discussion Paper 194 University of Kent at Canterbury, England: PSSRU.

Davies, B.P. and Challis, D.(1986) *Matching resources to needs in community care.* Aldershot: Gower.

Davies, B.P., Darton, R., and Goddard, M. (1987) *The effects of alternative targeting criteria and demand levels for the opportunity costs to the SSD of care in local authority homes.* Discussion Paper 484, University of Kent at Canterbury, England: PSSRU.

Dexter, M. and Harbert, W. (1983) *The Home Help Service.* London: Tavistock.

DHSS (Department of Health and Social Services) Social Services Inspectorate (1987) *From home help to home care: An analysis of policy, resourcing and service management.* London: DHSS.

Granneman, T.W., Grossman, J.B., and Millar Dunstan, S. (1986) *Differential impacts among subgroups of channelling enrollees.* Princeton, NJ: Mathematica Policy Research.

Griffiths, Sir R. (1988) *Community care: Agenda for action,* London: HMSO.

Hughes, S.L. (1988) 'Apples and oranges: A review of evaluations of community-based long-term care'. *Health Services Review* 20, 249–259.

Hunter, D., McKeganey, N., and Macpherson, I. (1988). *Care of the elderly: policy and practice.* Aberdeen: Aberdeen University Press.

Jansson, T. and Wallburg, E. (1988) *Care of the elderly in the Nordic countries: Costs, qualities, management.* Stockholm: Statskontoret, SAFAD.

Justice, D. *et al* (1988) *State long-term care reform: development of community care systems of six states.* Health Policy Studies. Washington D.C.: National Governors' Association Center for Policy Research.

Kane, R. (1988) 'The noblest experiment of them all. Learning from the national channelling evaluation'. *Health Services Research* 12, 189–198.

Kasper, J.D. (1990). 'Cognitive impairment among functionally limited elderly people in the community: Future considerations for long-term care policy'. *The Milbank Quarterly* 68, 81–110.

Kemper, P (1988) 'The evaluation of the national long-term care demonstration: Overview of the findings'. *Health Services Research* 23, 161–74.

Kemper, P. (1990) 'Case management agency systems of administering long-term care'. *The Gerontologist* 30, 817–824.

Kemper, P., Abblebaum, R., and Harrigan, M. (1987) 'Community care demonstrations: What have we learned?' *Health Care Financing Review* 8, 87–100.

Neill, J., Sinclair, I., Gorbach, P., and Williams, J. (1988) *A need for care: Elderly applicants for local authority homes.* Aldershot: Gower.

Netten, A. and Davies, B.P. (1990) 'The social production of welfare and consumption of social services'. *Journal of Public Policy* 10 (3) 331–334

The Pepper Commission (1990) US bi-partisan commission on comprehensive health care. A call for action: final report: US Government Printing Office, Washington DC.

Price Waterhouse (1991) *Caring for people: implementing community care: Purchase, commissioner and provider roles.* London: HMSO.

Pruger, R. (1987) *Making information work: The story of the Equity Project.* Berkeley, California: School of Social Welfare, University of California.

PSSRU (1992, forthcoming) *Community services and the social production of* welfare. Aldershot: PSSRU Studies Avebury / Gower.

Qureshi, H., Challis, D. and Davies, B.P. (1988) *Helpers in case-managed community care.* Aldershot: Gower.

Quine, L., and Pahl, J. (1985) 'Examining the causes of stress in families with mentally handicapped children'. *British Journal of Social Work* 15, 501–17.

Royal Commission on Local Government in England (1969) *Report of the Royal Commission on Local Government in England 1966–1969,* Cmnd 4040. London: HMSO.

Ruchlin, H.S., Morris, J.N., and Eggert, G.M. (1982A) 'Financing long-term care: A reply'. *New England Journal of Medicine* 306, 101–6.

Rutter, M., Tizard, J. and Whitmore, K. (1970) *Education health and behaviour.* London: Longman.

Seidl, F.W., Applebaum, R., Austin, C.D., and Mohoney, K.J. (1983) *Delivering in-home services to the aged and disabled: The Wisconsin experience.* Lexington, Mass: Lexington Books.

Sinclair, I. (1990) 'Residential care'. In Sinclair, I. Parker, R. Leat, D. and Williams, J. *The Kaleidoscope of Care,* London: HMSO.

Skellie, A., Dennis, L., Favor, F., Tudor, C., and Strauss, R. (1982) *Alternative health services project: Final report.* Atlanta, Georgia: Department of Medical Assistance.

Skellie, A., Mobley, G.M. and Coan, R.E. (1982) 'Cost-effectiveness of community-based long-term care: Current findings of Georgia's Alternative Health Services Project', *American Journal of Public Health* 72, 353–8.

Spector, W.D. (1991) 'Cognitive impatient and disruptive behaviours among community-based elderly persons: Implications for targeting long-term care'. *The Gerontologist* 31, 51–60.

Stewart, J.D. (1974) *The responsive local authority.* Tonbridge, Kent: Charles Knight.

Stewart, J. and Stoker, G. (1988) *From local administration to community government.* Fabian Research Series 331, London: Fabian Society.

Weissert, W., Cready, C., and Pawelak, J. (1988) 'The past and future of home and community-based long-term care'. *The Milbank Quarterly* 66, 309–88.

Index